To · Kathleen

# Discover the Secrets of Ageing Well and Staying Active

A must-read to uncover the benefits of 100% Natural Physiotherapy Treatments to maintain a healthy lifestyle -Essential reading for people Aged 40+

## By Tinashe (Nash) Dangarembizi

# Copyright

## © 2021 Tinashe Dangarembizi

Publisher: Tinashe Dangarembizi
**69 Bolton Road Kearsley BL4 8DB**

# About the Author

Tinashe (Nash) Dangarembizi is a highly qualified physiotherapist based in the United Kingdom. He is the proud founder of the rapidly growing *T4 Physio* Private Multiple Site Clinics situated in Manchester. *T4 Physio* serves a wide range of clientele, including individuals aged 40 and above. The ethos of *T4 Physio* is to assist individuals in staying active and independent using entirely natural treatments, thereby reducing inappropriate and unnecessary usage of pain medication.

Nash is also known as the "Physio for the stars" – he was head hunted to treat the BBC's Strictly Come Dancing professional dancers in the North West of England. During the off season of Strictly, Nash continues to offer physiotherapy treatments to the professional dancing stars. This has resulted in him treating more high prolife individuals and featuring in the Manchester Evening News and Bolton News.

Nash's clinics are the first micro-lab Physiotherapy clinics in the North West of England to own a revolutionary 3D Orthotic/Insoles prescribing machine. This means T4 Physio is able to provide top quality, long lasting, custom-made footwear accessories such as sandals, flip-flops, and T4 branded trainers. When it comes to minimising the risk of developing unwanted muscle tension, joint stiffness, and pain, Nash is obsessed with feet, and he is forever involved in footwear research and development projects. He is also evolving into a well-known business-man who is heavily involved with local charity work to serve his local community.

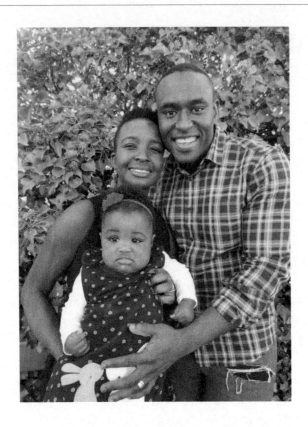

I dedicate this book to my beautiful wife Bernadette Dangarembizi and to Talia-Rose Tadisa Dangarembizi, my daughter. May this book inspire you to live a healthy abundant life, and thank you both for your unconditional love and support. For a solid upbringing I would like to give honor and praise to my parents Tiki and Sarudzai Dangarembizi and my grandmother Matilda Kaparadza. May this book be legacy to my family and anyone else who reads it.

# What Others are Saying

*Nash was on hand for Aljaz and I throughout our time training for Strictly Come Dancing. He was extremely professional and made us feel totally at ease to be around. Nash came to us whenever we were training and always tried to fit us in despite his already busy schedule. He helped prevent a lot of injuries from us dancing for 8hrs a day. Without him on hand I would have been in bits! I highly recommend Nash for any Physio needs and continue to use him when needed myself even though the show has finished.*

*Gemma Atkinson*

*I met Nash through the BBC Strictly Come Dancing crew and I have continued to receive treatment from you him because he is one of the best physios I have seen. I love coming to T4 Physio not only for the physio but the whole experience of having a drink and chatting to the T4 Physio team, it is such warm and friendly environment. I highly recommend a visit T4 Physio if you want to have an unforgettable physiotherapy experience.*

*Gorka Marquez*

*Extremely friendly, informative and considerate for my situation / condition. Was very helpful with suggestions on things I should consider OUTSIDE of the clinic to ensure that symptoms don't worsen when I dance. Nash was willing to travel to the dancing studio to offer his excellent physio services. I highly recommend him….top physio.*

*Oti Mabuse*

*I love coming to T4 Physio clinic for pre and post-fight physiotherapy/cryotherapy treatment. My favourite treatment is cryotherapy as this reduces swelling, improves metabolism and aids recovery after fight. The staff at the clinic are very friendly and I highly recommend T4 Physio Clinic to anyone with aches and pains.*

*Anthony Crolla*

*In preparation of my dancing competition, Nash offered excellent Sports Massage and Cryotherapy treatment. Such a friendly guy and make you feel at ease instantly. Great guy to be around and an excellent physio too. Thank you.*

*Karen Hauer*

# Introduction

Welcome. This book has been many years in the making, and as a new father navigating a recent COVID-normal, just like you, it's nice to have the space to share advice, tips, and to offer support. Underlying everything in the pages you're about to read is the fact that pain does not have to be part of your daily life. If you're struggling with chronic pain, or simply want to avoid doing so in the future, then this book is for you. As I stated at the beginning, much of the information you'll encounter throughout is a must read for individuals over 40 plus... so, I'll mostly be talking to you, in particular. However, if you're reading this and don't fall into that category, don't despair. A lot of the advice and tips you'll find here will benefit you, too. So if you're ready, let's get started on your life changing journey to a pain-free and active life!

The aim of this book is to highlight that "our health is our wealth, and our wealth is our health". Take a moment to reflect on that. Isn't that powerful? On his deathbed, Steve Jobs famously said the following:

*What is the world's most expensive bed? The hospital bed. At this time, lying on the hospital bed and remembering all my life, I realise that all the accolades and riches of which I was once so proud, have become insignificant with my imminent death.*

This is an incredibly resonating quote. How often is it that we become entangled in things that have nothing to do with our quality of life or health? How often do we lose sight of how to take care of ourselves?

This simple quote sums up the importance of our health being our true wealth. It underlines the fact that we have to take care of our health – the rest will follow and pales in comparison. As such, it is paramount that we look within ourselves and ask whether we're doing enough. Are we maintaining a healthy lifestyle? Eating well? Staying active and mobile? Are we living the lives we were meant to live? If the answers to these questions are difficult to come by, don't worry. It's because of this very reason that I wrote this book, and it's exactly why you're in precisely the right place. I want you to enjoy a healthful life – pain free!

So with this in mind, and as the old cliché goes, "life begins at 40". In fact, this may very well be the age at which you start reconsidering your habits and lifestyle – this may be the age at which one starts to value health and where one is willing to stay fit and well. I see this in my clinics every day. And that's a large part of why I wrote this book! I want to encourage you to become "patient experts" in managing chronic aches/pains in a healthful way… with minimal medication usage. Health in abundance!

Pain or joint stiffness/tension is something you're probably dealing with. If you've picked up this book, my guess is that you're currently living with chronic pain that's holding you back from living the life you deserve. The pain is getting in the way of your relationships, your dreams, and your health – it's stealing the happiness from your life. So I encourage you to make a stand, right now. Choose to manage the pain, choose to change your life, and choose a healthful way to maintain a great qualify of life. I'm here to help.

This book's main aim is to help you understand how to manage chronic pain via the proactive application of activity, that is, through revamping your lifestyle to incorporate healthful activity and mobility.

**Discover the Secrets of Ageing Well and Staying Active**

Longevity is, after all, powered by mobility, and moving your body – correctly – is a sure-fire way of getting back to a pain-free life. In view of this, I will also address some of the commonly held myths around staying active, and I'll provide practical tools and proven advice to help you overcome common misconceptions about exercise. At the end of the day, I want you to get moving and I'm here to help you do just that!

Before we jump into all of that, I'd like to remind you that for every barrier there is in your life, there is a solution you can employ to overcome it. For every roadblock you encounter on your journey to health and a pain free life, there is a way you can jump over. Life gives us obstacles to make us stronger – embrace them, learn from them, and grow stronger because of them.

As we move further into this book, you'll learn a lot about ways in which you can improve your mobility and health in order to manage chronic pain effectively. Before we get there, though, we need to think about precisely why pain can get exacerbated or feel an impossible mountain to overcome. The uncanny thing about pain is, is that is seems to stem from mysterious places – from daily habits, incorrect choices, or repetitive physical stress. You'd be surprised how few injuries truly result from serious trauma like a fall or accident! So, let's take a look at the less considered ways that pain can take hold in your life. Why?

Well, knowing the root cause always gets you closer to solving the problem  I would like to start by highlighting the foundation of the body which includes bones, tendons, ligaments and soft tissue that make up the musculoskeletal system of the human body.

The word musculoskeletal can be broken down into muscles, bones, tendons, ligaments, and all these elements are designed to work together in harmony and act as a hinge to support the body's weight and help us to move. It is within this framework that all body functions operate; these include the vital organs like the heart, lungs, and brain. Unfortunately, it can also be the same framework that injuries, diseases, and the ageing process stem from due to number of controllable and uncontrollable factors. The good news is that, in most cases, we can keep the musculoskeletal system strong as we age, hereby staying active and enjoying a high quality life.

Let us start with the four common risk factors that can increase the chances of developing musculoskeletal diseases or general aches/pains. In this context, a risk factor is anything that is likely to increase the chances of developing an injury or a condition.

## Poor Posture

To a physiotherapist like me, posture means everything! But I have a secret to share with you… it should mean everything to you, too! Poor posture can contribute to muscular and joint aches/pains. So much so in some cases that arthritis can flare up, muscles can overcompensate causing joint pain, and a host of other similarly painful scenarios can develop.
Yet, what is posture in the first place? And why is it so important? Well, posture can simply be defined as the ability of the body to sustain a position for a time period using the correct muscles and least energy when standing, sitting, or moving.

Phew, a mouthful, right? Posture is really just the way your body responds to poses – whether correctly or incorrectly – and as a consequence, the way your muscles react to this.

As such, if you suffer from poor posture, it's very likely that your muscles will start to ache, your joints will cause you discomfort, and everyday movements may become strained. Over time, poor posture will most likely give way to chronic pain, and in some severe cases, body dysmorphia – a hunched back, limp, or slumped shoulder, may in some cases be due to a lifetime of incorrect posture.

More than this, though, poor posture can give rise to an entirely new host of problems – from back pain through to hip pain, incorrect posture stands as one of the main reasons so many of my clients saw it fit to see me. Correct the posture… manage and potentially eradicate the pain.

I'll be giving you a lot more information on poor posture through this book, but if you ever catch yourself slouching and maintaining poor posture for prolonged periods (usually for longer than 20-30 minutes at a time) then you might want to address it accordingly. This will minimise the risk of developing aches and pains in your joints/muscles.

## Sedentary Lifestyle

In this day and age many people live a sedentary lifestyle, all of which can contribute to poor posture, thereby increasing the risk of developing muscle stiffness. These mundane sedentary tasks may include desk/couch-based work, travelling to and from meetings, or prolonged driving which can increase the likelihood of developing obesity and cardiovascular diseases on top of chronic pain. Also, as I write this, many of you reading this may be working from home due to the COVID-19 epidemic and the Lockdown regulations implemented by the government.

Of course, this scenario means there is an influx of kitchen-desk offices, attic based conference rooms, and clandestine sofa time… all of which can wreak havoc on your posture. Please keep a look out for this – get up and stretch!

It is important to know that, as we age, muscles and their flexibility start to reduce slightly: this can affect the body's ability to maintain posture for prolonged periods, thereby resulting in poor posture and muscle tension. The answer? Get moving! More on that later.

How do you move… is it right or wrong?

Do you remember all those times your parents or friends used to say "don't lift that box!". Do you think you ought to have listened?
So many of the injuries I encounter in my clinics are as a result of incorrect lifts, or as we call them in the physiotherapy world, poor manual handling. Whether you're lifting a box, a toddler, or a dumbbell, the premise remains the same: never allow your center of gravity to be too far away from the weight itself, and never, ever lift with your back. Always use your legs to drive through into the weight.

My 8 month old daughter, Talia-Rose, is excellent at demonstrating the perfect squatting technique: she bends her legs to lower her body to floor in order to play with her toys. This is partly because she will lose her balance if she doesn't squat correctly.

Learning this type of technique can take time, especially as we pick-up bad habits as we get older or become lazy! Remember, it is crucial that you're aware of the risk of improper manual handling: from torn muscles, to slipped discs and a whole host of other issues, lifting weights without proper posture and technique can result in serious pain.

Don't worry, though, I'm going to walk you through how to approach these situations later on, but for now, please know that you need to think about how you're lifting heavy objects. If you're not aware of the long-term effects of incorrect manual handling, your daily life with be affected: from picking up shopping, to hauling a suitcase across the airport, life will become a lot harder.

If you're reading this and have already experienced this pain first hand, please don't give in – keep reading, there is a way out of your pain.

## Reduced Fitness

I can see you rolling your eyes – how in the world can reduced fitness levels be causing you pain? Surely the runners, long-jumpers, and snowboarders are the ones most likely to be in pain, right?

Well, no, not really. Fitness levels are a fairly good indicator of how much activity you do, and if you're not doing any then your muscles cannot maintain their mass or strength – they shorten, become stiff, and lose their ability to correctly support your joints, thereby causing increased – and eventually, chronic – pain.

Of course, as a result of immobility obesity and issues related to bearing to much weight can surface. Pain is, sadly, one of the most common side effects of dramatic weight gain. It's a viscous circle: no movement, more weight, more pain. The circle needs to be broken, and the only way to do so is to make a truly proactive choice related to your health.

I'll walk you through what I mean in more detail later on in the book, but for now, bear this in mind: in the UK, the general weekly exercise recommendation for adults is at least 150 minutes of moderately intense activity a week, or alternately, 75 minutes of high intensity activity with at least 2 days of strength training a week. Sound a bit much?

Well, the good news is that physical activities don't need to be boring. They can be anything you enjoy doing, like Zumba, dog walking, dancing, swimming, or many other things. It's about what suits you – you just need to make the decision to try.

In fact, normal daily activities such cooking, cleaning, DIY, gardening, or physical activities are also great ways to improve balance, especially for individuals that are 70+. Any type of activity makes a difference! The key thing to remember about muscles is that you can lose them if you do not use them… and it is quicker to lose muscle strength than to gain it. So, make it fun, set goals, and get moving!

# Poor Diet/Nutrition

Pain and nutrition are linked? Oh yes! In fact, what you put into your body has a direct effect on what it puts out. If you eat fast food every day, your body will suffer, you'll feel pains in your chest, and eventually you might suffer from muscular or cardiovascular breakdowns and diseases. Happily, the same principle applies the other way around, too! If you eat better food, your body will start functioning like a well-oiled machine – it will be so much better at managing chronic pain, your muscles will get the proper nutrients to support the body, and you'll find yourself left with more energy and vitality than ever before. And the best part? Your body will be able to stave off future injury and pain so much better!

There is an ongoing debate about the best diet/nutrition plan to lose weight and gain muscle, yet it is sad how much misinformation is being disseminated out there. Just remember, life is all about moderation – eat enough protein, good fats, vegetables, and carbs.
Avoid processed foods in so far as possible, and give sugar a miss if you can. Drink enough water and make sure you're well hydrated throughout the day. Changing your diet is about altering your lifestyle – make sure your choices are sustainable, healthful, and nutritious. Find out more on this throughout the book.

So, there you have it: I've outlined the 4 most important factors when it comes to increased chronic pain and unhealthy lifestyles. We can all be affected by these factors, but it is incredibly important to know that each of them can be altered and changed – we need only make the choice to do so.

If you're ready to make the changes needed, then I invite you to continue reading. It's time to end chronic pain and to learn how to manage it effectively in order to live the life you deserve.

As we move further into this book, we'll look at regions of the body where chronic pain is most common; we'll look at how we can manage pain in those regions, and I'll also offer you tips on how to manage pain and continuously improve your lifestyle so as to lead a healthful, happy life.

# Chapter 1

# Feet:  The Foundation of the Body

If you have ever stubbed your big toe against the corner of a table, then you will know that your body will come to a standstill to attend to the pain/discomfort. The reason for this is because our feet matter, and they do play an important role in the body. Chronic foot pain can be just as bad as chronic back pain, so the management of foot pain is crucial in achieving a happy life. Luckily, there is a way, and if you're one of the millions of people out there struggling with daily, debilitating foot pain, don't worry! This chapter exposes the importance of feet, addresses footwear, and explains the normal walking pattern to minimise injuries. By the end of it, you'll see a light at the end of the foot-pain tunnel, and my hope is that you'll get to your feet and make the choices to access the pain free life you deserve. There is a lot to learn in this chapter, so let's begin....

My passion for feet started after treating one of the BBC Strictly Come Dancing Stars who sustained an ankle injury during the show from dancing in heels. Thankfully I managed to treat her symptoms and reduce the stiffness and pain just in time for her live performance on TV.

Prior to this I had not really treated many dancers in the clinics, therefore I was not enlightened to the fact that very high heels were part of the dancing fashion.
My job was to treat the ankle sprain as a result of the intense training required to perform in the show while wearing heels. Talk about feeling the pressure, not only was I star-struck from treating my first celebrity client, but I had only 3 weeks to make sure she was able to continue with the dancing competition while wearing high heels during the performance.

Miraculously, though, I managed to treat the dancer and taped the ankle to ensure she was able to dance in heels throughout the show. Needless to say I was delighted that the dancer managed to recover from the injury and that she progressed to the later stages of the show. In hindsight, this was the first time I really understood that our feet are the foundations of the body as well as why supportive footwear is important when it comes to minimizing the risk of injury. Feet can be like Marmite – yeast extract - you either love it or you hate it. Whatever your views on feet may be, the truth is that they do play an important role in the body. In fact, they have one of the most important jobs there is: they support your body like the foundation under a house. Worth taking care of then, right?

The 26 bones found in each foot are supported by ligaments, tendons, and muscles; they allow us to stand, walk, or run, and they allow us to move fluidly and unlike almost any other living being on Earth. Your feet need looking after! One fairly positive outcome of this terrible COVID-19 pandemic is that more and more people have taken to spending time outdoors: from cycling, to walking, to running, more and more people are doing activities – most of which involve their feet!
Yet it's not all good new, I'm afraid. Sadly, there has been a fairly significant increase in lower body injuries, such as runner's knee and plantar fasciitis. Why? The number one culprit is incorrect footwear, followed very closely by improper posture, running on hard surfaces, and perhaps a general ignorance of the environment. Whatever the reason, though, taking care of your feet is a good place to start when avoiding things like movement-related injuries.

Not everyone has the same type of foot: we may encounter flat feet with shallow arches, or higher feet with taller arches – each beautiful and each valuable. So it is vitally important to wear footwear with adequate support where possible. This is to maintain the foot's natural arch and to minimise foot disease such as plantar fasciitis. The latter is a disease that targets the tendons in the foot – visit my website www.t4physio.co.uk for more information on this and other foot related issues.

If, however, you tend to shop for style over functionality, then it might be time to make a change – especially if you suffer from foot, back, hip, or leg pain. One way of doing so is to look into bespoke orthotics. No, not braces! Orthotics are insoles designed specifically for the shape of your foot – they offer optimal support and ensure that you're able to maintain a good gait when walking. In other words, your muscles are offered the support needed for them to function optimally, thereby eradicating pain. If you're a gym fanatic, for example, a bespoke insole or orthotic can also help you to squat effectively and reduce the risk of heel lift if prescribed with the correct home exercise program. But don't stop there! Whether you're a hiker, walker, runner, or keen roller-skate enthusiast, orthotics will help increase good form and posture during your chosen activity, thereby helping you avoid injury. This is a key step in pain management, too!

## What type of footwear is best for me?

The shoes we wear on our feet are a great way to protect them from unsafe environments: they offer support, help us to walk or run better, and they minimise the risk of muscle or joint injuries. You never thought your Jimmy Choo's did so much, did you? Well, maybe they don't. Shoes can actually do us just as much harm as good, especially when we don't take into account the amount of support they really offer. In fact, an incorrect shoe can cause all of the very same issues they're meant to prevent!

The bottom line? Your footwear should give you adequate support and protection without causing long-term damage or injuries.

Personally, I see so many foot problems stem from inadequate footwear. We live in a world that takes fashion more seriously than comfort sometimes. The corporate world we live in almost always forces us to wear formal working shoes, the design of which often leaves little to be desired in terms of support. This has to be addressed – in fact, making a change here, in something you do practically every single day, can make a huge difference in your experience of chronic pain. Trainers such a Nike or Sketchers tend to be much more comfortable in addition to supplying adequate heel and middle arch support. When compared to standard office shoes, there really is little comparison. Now, I'm not saying rush out and buy Nike – no. What I am saying, though, is be sure to make an informed decision about the footwear you purchase. I do see more and more people wearing trainers with their office attire, so there is an awakening as to the importance of looking after your feet. Be encouraged by this and make your own change.

Pointy shoes, in particular, can alter gait by pressuring the big toe to turn. This can have devastating results. When one's walking pattern is affected for a long time there is an increased risk of being exposed to ground force reactions, that is, shocks running up through the foot, into the ankle and joints, and then through to the knee and hip joints. Long term, this can lead to debilitating chronic pain, the results of which can be devastating. If the joint pain and/or stiffness is left untreated, then it might result in degenerative joint issues such as Osteoarthritis. In medical terms, "osteo" means bones, and "arthritis" means inflammation/swelling and stiffness in the joints. Put those two together and you're in for a lot of unnecessary pain – all of which can potentially be lessened by the proper footwear being worn.

Now, let's be clear here, I am certainly not saying that if you wear pointy or narrow shoes you will get Osteoarthritis. What I am saying, however, is that it is a risk factor that that type of footwear exposes you to risk, the results of which may have serious repercussions later on in life.

So, look after your feet. If you do that, they'll certainly look after you: it's what they're designed to do. They are the foundation of your body... and you wouldn't build your house on sand, would you? Turn to chapter 10 to find out about a simple solution to make sure you give your feet the support they deserve, all without needing to buy new shoes.

## The Basics of Walking

It might be hard to imagine now, but can you recall the first time you took your first step? If you can, that's pretty amazing!

On a serious note, though, I bet taking that first step was not easy. I actually think it must have been like learning to walk on the moon – you had to implement a completely new set of muscles, activate different senses, and generally find balance you didn't even know you had. Don't be too hard on yourself, though. The reason why walking is initially difficult is because it is actually a very complex process.

Do you remember that I mentioned good posture is essential in maintaining great health and a pain free life overall? Well, gait, and by association feet, go hand-in-hand when it comes to this part of health. But what is gait anyway? Gait, in simple terms, is the way we walk. So, it's a good idea to come to grips with the complexity of walking. Why? So that you have a better idea of how to improve your own gait moving forward so as to mitigate chronic pain in your life. Pain or injury to your feet can cause a cascade of changes up the body causing havoc as I uncover this book reveals how chapter by chapter from toe to head.

Not because I want to teach you how to walk, here is a step by step break down of a normal walking pattern to reduce the risk of injury/pain to the foot/ankle but potentially to the rest of the body.

We will start with the heel strike phase, and this is exactly "what it says on the tin". Yes, that's right. A heel strike occurs when the heel of the foot touches the ground first for a short period of time, thereafter lifting up again. This is important as it sets the walking pattern in motion.
Interestingly, the muscles responsible for this phase are your lower leg and buttocks muscles. If done incorrectly, the hip is directly affected, as well as the knees and overall gait. It is essential that you note your own heel strike in order to assess it for correction. If you're unsure, contact a qualified, hands-on physiotherapist for advice and help.

The second step involves the muscles underneath the foot; they act as shock absorbers from the ground force reactions, thereby causing the inside of the foot to roll into a position called "pronation". Pronation is when the foot/ankle joint turns slightly inwards which is good as this allows the foot to propel forward to the next phase. It not uncommon to see patients at the clinic with over-pronation that is, a state whereby the foot rolls in too much on the instep thus resulting in ankle/foot overloading and potentially injuries to foot/ankle and potentially compensation to the rest of the joints above.

Complicated jargon, maybe, but this simply means that the door is opened for foot/ankle injuries. During this phase of the walking pattern, it is not uncommon to identify weakness/stiffness of the lower leg and buttock muscles, all of which can affect the foot position and weight transfer as the foot connects with the ground upon treading.

It is very important, therefore, that you are aware of the way in which your foot rolls upon striking the ground. It is in this second phase, perhaps more than the others, where we see the benefits of orthotics really come into play as explained in chapter 10.

This next phase is a crucial phase in the walking cycle, as it is where the body faces the most risk to injury to the foot/ankle. Here, the body will only be supported by one single leg as the other leg starts to swing forward which means you need the muscles above the foot such as your thigh muscles and buttocks to be strong the stop the foot collapsing. If you're naturally flat footed you can potentially develop foot disease such as bunions due to increased ground force reactions that might cause joint(s) pain in the lower body. If you have a high arch then you might predispose to ankle injury in this phase of the walking pattern. Needless to say if you wear unsupported shoes like heels then you might just be asking for trouble.

The penultimate phase is the toe-off phase which starts as the heel leaves the ground and as the body weight is transferred forward; the knee also bends slightly at this stage. These movements are closely followed by the toe off phase, that is, when the toes leaves the ground.

If we think back to my earlier discussion regarding narrow and pointy footwear, it is interesting to note that some people don't actually have a toe phase due to prolonged use of these types of shoes. Their big left toe points west and the right toe points east so instead of using their big toes to push off of the ground, they use the side of the big toe instead hence bunion injury can occur.

If left untreated, this causes mechanical foot issues that can lead to muscle imbalances and foot disease, and compensation reaction to the rest of the joints and muscles above the foot.

The last phase before the cycle is repeated is called the swing phase, so named in preparation of the heel strike phase coming up again. In this phase, the muscles at the back of leg help to control the movement of the foot as it prepares for the next heel strike. Again, improper form in this phase could lead to a gait that may give rise to pain down the line.

And there you have it: a 'normal' walking pattern in a nutshell. Again, the reason I outlined this for you is to draw your attention to the importance of proper form in your gait – not displaying proper form in your posture, particularly in your tread, could lead to potentially debilitating problems.

A walking patterns seems simple, yet is masterfully complex. Many of the lower-body injuries we encounter in my clinic are as a direct result of improper form during the walking cycle. To find more about how a poor footwear, abnormal walking pattern and foot mechanics can cause havoc to the rest of the body then Chapter 10 is waiting for you.

The aim of this first chapter was to highlight that the foundation of the body has to be properly assessed and scrutinised as issues with foot mechanics, normal walking pattern and even footwear could be the root cause of your ongoing aches and pains if left untreated for a prolonged period. It also highlights how the body should never be treated in isolation as how you present on the treatment table could be total different to when you start moving.

Therefore, simple changes in your lifestyle, minor correction to foot function may go beyond your wildest dreams and be the difference between keeping active or not. The root cause of pain can, at times, be elusive, yet when it comes to lower-body chronic pain, a good place to start looking is at the feet.

At *T4 Physio* clinics, we aim to give you the answers you need, the advice you are looking for, and a way to help mitigate and treat the ongoing pain you're dealing with. I hope this chapter has given you some insight into the important role the foot has to play in chronic pain, but if you have any questions or concerns, I invite you to visit my website and book a FREE 15 minutes consultation with a foot specialist to learn more. Simply follow the link, here: www.t4physio.co.uk/contact. I'm here to help and we can send you a free Foot Guide upon request.

Now that we've delved into the intricacies of the foot, it's time to move up the body to the knee in order to see how you can start managing pain overall. In this way, I aim to give you an overview of how pain may function in the body, thereby giving you some idea of how you can start managing it and living a pain free life. Ready? Let's jump straight in.

# Chapter 2

## Knees: A Well Oiled Knee is a gift as you age!

As the heading of this chapter explains, we're looking at the knees next. I bet you've not given them much thought, have you? In fact, the knee is one of the most underappreciated parts of the body whilst, ironically, it may well be one of the parts that work the hardest!

Your knees are the strongest hinge joints you have, and yet their strength doesn't dampen their flexibility. In fact, their unique flexibility and strength underscores their invaluable place in your overall body's health. Why are they so important, though? Well, on the one hand they facilitate the streamlined movement of your lower legs and thighs. And you know what that means, right? A healthy posture! On the other hand, too, they act as shock absorbers: they take the brunt of each step you take, the pressure of which can be immense if you're not careful.

Which brings us to the core of this chapter: knee pain. If you're like one of the millions of people around the globe who suffer from knee pain, then you know that doing simple things such as gardening, kneeling, walking the dog, or even getting into bed can be an ordeal. Knee pain can be unbearable and can truly steal your joy if left unaddressed. So, it really should be avoided at all costs.

As I mentioned, your knee joint is particularly vulnerable to pain because it takes the full weight of your body each time you stand, step, or sit. This pressure is increased exponentially when you squat, run or jump. Now, don't get me wrong – you cannot avoid activity as a means to avoid knee pain. In fact, if you are going that route, then you might find yourself worse-off … knees need to move! It's how you move that matters. Let me reiterate – if you're currently suffering from knee plain, please know that avoidance of activity is not the cure. It is important to remain active so as to assist with the healing of your knee and to keep your knee fit and healthy. This will prevent future injuries from occurring. If you are injured, daily activities should be modified for a few days in order to enable movement whilst allowing the pain settle.

In this chapter, then, I'd like to look at the knee and why "well oiled" knees are so important. I want to focus on the knee because so many of my own patients suffer from knee pain, many of whom could have avoided their suffering by taking the proper precautions early on. My goal is to give you hope that your chronic knee pain can be managed, to give you the tools to do so, and to get you back to living an active, gleeful lifestyle. Buckle up and let's dive into this chapter.

At the risk of losing you at the get go, let's start with the boring, basic science of the knee joint and get that out of the way first. Come on… this stuff is important! The longest bone in the body is the femur. Your thigh muscles surround this bone and together they join with the lower leg bones – known as the tibia and fibula – to make up the knee joint. Still with me? Trust me, knowing what it is plays a massive role in understanding how it works. And then? Less pain!

So, sitting in front of the knee is the patella, and although this bone is small, it plays a very important role in making sure we can bend and straighten the knee smoothly. Finally, inside the knee joint there is fluid known as the synovial fluid; this lubricates the knee joint, thereby enabling streamlined movement.

If you've not gone through the coming-of-age dissection in biology at college, then shuffle on over to the kitchen. If you are a meat lover like I am, then look no further than the chicken thighs in your fridge for a deeper understanding of the knee. On the fowl's thigh, look out for the top part of the bone covered in a white slippery-textured substance. That's called cartilage, and just like Chicken Little, you have it too. In fact, you have a few of these cartilage formations around the bones that make up the knee joint.

Now that you've got some idea of what the knee joint looks like, let's turn to why it could be placed under stress which, ultimately, causes you pain. In the first instance, the synovial fluid in your knee reduces and slowly thickens with age, thereby causing "early morning knee" stiffness. It's really called this! When you get out of bed in the morning your knee might be stiff and it may take you a few minutes to walk or stretch in order to warm up the knee joint. The truth is, the older we get the less "well-oiled" our joints are. We don't have the ability to sail through the day without feeling a bit of wear-and-tear on our knees anymore. Age affects the cartilage, too, I'm afraid. We know that cartilage assists the knee when moving, but as we age it tends to dry out, thereby causing extra abrasion in the knee and – you guessed it – pain.

To be clear, though, this is absolutely normal as you increase in age, and even knowing about it cannot prevent it from happening. However, we can delay the ageing process by making sure the muscles, ligaments, fluids, tendons and bones around the knee joint remain strong. This is very, very important. In order to maximise our overall physical function and to maintain excellent quality of life as we age, we have to take care of our knees.

I bet you didn't know that the knee joint affects practically every part of your body, did you? Your back pain could be as a result of your knee, your neck pain, too... in fact, I wouldn't be surprised if your earache was! In all seriousness, though, your knee joint has the ability to seriously debilitate other areas of your body. My patients are always really surprised when they attend the clinic for knee treatment and I start assessing the joints above and below the knee. They frequently – and frantically – ask me: "What does this have to with my knee, Nash?" I smile and always explain the following: the knee shares some muscles with the hip, whilst some of the foot muscles overlap with the knee muscles. Ultimately, this means that, if the hip or foot/ankle muscles are in a bad state, then this may cause knee pain... and vice versa. Everything is linked! That's what makes the body so incredible.

As you'll recall, I drew your attention to the importance of feet and a normal walking pattern in the first chapter. Well, if those two aren't at their optimal form, then you may very well experience nagging knee pain that just will not go away. It may well leave you in pieces and not in peace!

So, am I saying that the muscle imbalances in the hip and foot can affect the knee? Correct! In fact, I'll share a secret with you: understanding the body holistically – as an interconnected whole – is a concept that separates experienced and skilled physiotherapists from junior, less experienced ones. Turn to Chapter 10 of this book to find how the body's unwanted tension can travel from the feet up to the upper body.

The ability and skill to discern whether patients with knee pain should be given treatment for the knee via a holistic approach to the body could be the difference between lifelong pain and a much-needed reprieve from suffering. It could very well mean you can pick your grandkids up rather than watching from afar. Please remember this when approaching a physiotherapist – the entire body is interlinked, so your pain is hardly ever a localised issue, especially when it comes to the knee.

To be truthful, I treat many patients that have been suffering with knee pain for years prior to seeing me. Their mistake? Their previous therapists didn't approach their knee pain holistically; they kept going to the therapists time after time yet experienced limited improvement.

I don't want that to be you. So, my hope is to give you the tools to discern the correct treatment for your knee despite you, yourself, lacking medical knowledge, or at least to give you a basic understanding of what may be contributing to your pain so as to correctly mitigate the discomfort. Here are a few major contributing factors that I see at my clinic, all of which typically cause knee pain:

# Age

Imagine this, from the day you're born you start using your joints for movement and support, so if you're 40 years old then you have spent 350 400 hours of your life using your joints! That is an incredible amount of time! Now, I don't know about you, but that's a lot of hours... wear and tear is inevitable. No wonder age is one of the biggest contributing factors to knee pain, right? The good news is there is a way to mitigate the risks associated with the ageing process. As we move through this book, I'll be delving into the following advice at various stages during these pages, but all-in-all the information below is invaluable to any body part, especially those ones in pain.

So, how can you minimise the stress on joints, especially on your knees, particularly when you can't slow down the ageing process? Nope, it's definitely NOT Botox. If you do take Botox, though, there's no judgement here. I am, however, talking about utilising 100% natural treatments such as exercises, a balanced diet, and meditation. Of course, age is just a number yet it is a very significant one... if you don't believe me, then check your insurance premium as you age! Remember, though, you don't have to feel or act your age if you take care of your body and look after it.

It is important to remember that what you do in your 40's will have significant repercussions in your 50s. And, what you do in your 50's will most definitely effect you in your 60's. So, what you do in your 60's... you catch my drift, right? Every single choice you make now directly affects your future self. Wouldn't it be wise to make the right decision, then?

Now, if you are female then you may be familiar with the term "menopause". Firstly, let me point out that menopause is NOT a dirty word; it is a natural biological process that marks the end of the menstrual cycle. This means that the body ceases to produce eggs for fertilisation. Think of this not so much as an end but as a chance to really make some healthful changes in your life. You might very well be thinking "what has this got to do with my knee, Nash?" Well, a lot more than you may have realised, actually! Alongside the many other effects of menopause – hot flashes and hormonal imbalances – this mid-life transformation can be a game changer when it comes to weak bones (osteoporosis) and weight gain.

Let's delve into osteopersosis for a minute, since it's often an age-related ailment. As I mentioned in Chapter 1, the word "osteo" refers to bone, whilst the term "porosis" means insecure or weak. So therefore, their combination, that is, "osteoporosis", means a weakening of the bones, the result of which is, yes, you guessed it…. pain – particularly when it comes to your knees. Knee joints are especially vulnerable to the effects of osteoporosis, as they have to carry the weight of the torso and are responsible for transferring the body's weight through the leg and foot much like a bridge would do. In fact, they literally bridge the lower and upper body.

The bottom line really is that strength exercises are incredibly important for knee health, especially for women. These types of exercises work the muscles and bones in such a way as to fortify and strengthen them against age related degeneration. You can find out more about the benefits of exercises in Chapter 6, as well as the benefits of Physiotherapy Treatment in Chapter 9.

If you've ever wondered why infants are encouraged to jump up and down, wonder no more: it's to encourage bone growth. So, as we age it is crucial to safely perform high impact exercises and weight training to facilitate and maintain strong bones, much like a baby eases into it when it's young. Furthermore, calcium levels tend to deplete with age, so mitigating the effect of this is crucial.

A tip? Make sure you're taking adequate vitamin D supplements, that you're enjoying the sunshine, taking some good fat capsules, drinking plenty of water, and eating a balanced diet. All this, as well as making healthful choices along the way, plays a major part in giving the body all the nutrients it needs to keep the knee and other joints working smoothly. This will help you avoid hip replacements and general joint diseases, too!

## Weight Gain

Now, let's talk about weight gain. Controversial? Well, maybe, but it plays a big role in knee pain. In fact, most female patients I treat suffer from extra discomfort due to a little extra weight, yet they often suffer in silence whether due to fear of judgement or embarrassment. The thing is, everyone goes through this – and if you're a female dealing with menopause, then it's even more natural. There is no reason to be embarrassed – and if you're suffering because of it then something needs to change.

I'm going to chat to you about why getting older – and going through menopause – can cause weight gain. Before then, though, I want to be brutally honest. If you've gained weight due to menopause, please don't use this as a way to 'accept' the weight and not to change it. Being overweight is not only unhealthily in the long term, but can exasperate your knee pain and potentially cause other ailments, too. It's not embarrassing, but it needs to be looked into.

The two major hormones affected by menopause are oestrogen and progesterone – they deplete with age. Without going into a chemistry lecture here (because that would be boring), let me touch on the role of these two hormones, particularly when it comes to weight gain. Oestrogen is known as the sex hormone and it has different functions in the body, from controlling puberty development to underscoring bone strength. As such, it is the reduction of oestrogen in the body that increases the chances of developing osteoporosis. That aside, if left untreated, low levels of oestrogen can interrupt the normal function of the thyroid, too. And here is where weight gain comes into play. The interruption of thyroid function leads to an altered metabolic rate, thereby resulting in an increased conversion of carbohydrates into fats, as well as an increased appetite for sugars. The result? Weight gain.

On the other hand, progesterone helps the body to prepare for pregnancy by getting the uterus ready. So, when this hormone depletes, as happens during menopause, it results in headaches, migraines, and mood swings, to list but a few. The result? Stress eating in most cases.

Oftentimes, women may turn to hormone replacement therapy. The use of HRT sees the replacement of these two common hormones, the result of which can mitigate the effects of menopause. In the United Kingdom, HRT can be accessed via the General Practitioner (GP). Should you require more information please contact your local GP practice.

Lower levels of these two hormones can have serious effects not just on your mental health, but on your physical wellbeing, too. Though weight gain is a general side effects of menopause, it does not mean it has to be an inevitable one: you can make a positive change, the result of which will mean less knee pain, a more active lifestyle, and a quality of life you deserve.

As we move into the later chapters of this book, I will discuss in detail the benefits of regular exercise. For now, though, try to incorporate regular activity into your life, as the endorphins – a peptide as powerful as morphine – increase a sense of contentment, happiness, and fulfilment. And that can only be good, right?

## Obesity

Speaking of gaining weight, we now turn to the extreme result of weight gain: obesity. Gaining weight and being obese are two different things – the former presents a shift in weight, whilst the latter refers to a body mass index well beyond what is healthy. Obesity and pain are directly linked, and if you're currently within a dangerous BMI range then you'll know what I'm referring to. Losing weight is the single most important thing you can do to ease the pain.

To be honest, I'm shocked by how many of the patients who attend my clinic don't know about the direct correlation between obesity and knee pain. I want to be clear – your knee pain will always be a problem unless your weight is addressed. Physiotherapy can help, but the strain placed on your knee joint will always prevent your knee from recovering correctly.

Let me try to put this into context for you. Imagine that you are a Mercedes Benz and you constantly drive around carrying large suitcases packed with items such as clothes and shoes everywhere you go. Eventually, the shock absorbers may squeak and the tires may run down, right? Well, this exactly what constantly carrying extra body weight does to your body: it weighs it down and increases the risk of injury and cardiovascular disease immensely. To put it into perspective, when it comes to knee pain, carrying an extra 4.5 kilos automatically adds an extra 10-20 kilos of pressure onto your knees. Ultimately, this increases the risk of developing osteoarthritis or worsening any pre-existing joint related ailments. It can only end badly.

Later in this book I talk about diet – if you're currently suffering from obesity-related pain, please read my advice. You deserve the quality of life you dream of.

## Poor Exercise Technique/Form

So, we now know about weight gain, obesity, and hormonal fluctuations during menopause, but what about exercise?

I am a big gym fan, and as I am writing this the gyms have been closed for 3 months due to the Covid-19 pandemic... I'm heartbroken, really. Exercise is so important, and it's my wish for you that you feel excited about becoming active, healthy, and mobile! When it comes to knee pain, specifically, doing exercise is essential. Here's the thing, though, not all exercises are equal, and as the knee joint is so intricate, it's very, very important to do the right exercises to strengthen it. Let's run through a few incorrect exercises I see in the gym all too often.

You don't need to be an Olympic weight lifter to know that squatting exercises – with or without weights – sure look easy. It's deceptive, though! Squatting requires a very specific technique so as to ensure you don't hurt your knees or back. If done incorrectly, you can easily overload the knee muscles/tendons resulting in knee injury and pain. I'm not going to run through what a correct squat looks like, here, Instead, I want to give you my top 5 tips for minimising knee pain when you squat:

1. Stretch your lower leg muscles at least 3-4 times a week.
2. Make sure your knees do not go over your toes.
3. Wear orthotics or lifting shoes if your heels lift from the ground.
4. Turn your feet out slightly.
5. Keep your upper body as straight as possible.


Squatting is just one form of strengthening activity, but I am definitely an advocate for all forms of exercises. I'd like to be clear, though... exercise is fantastic when it done correctly.
The COVID-19 pandemic has left more and more people with exercise related injuries... why? Well, YouTube doesn't really tell you what the correct form for a squat, plank, or burpee is, right?

All too many of the patients I've seen recently have undergone an injury – particularly knee injuries – that could otherwise have been avoided. Now, it is fantastic that people can exercise at home using YouTube videos or Joe Wicks exercise clips, but with a virtual instructor there is an increased risk of poor technique. This can, in turn, result in knee joint pain and other injuries. Please be careful and always consult a physiotherapist if you're unsure about your technique.

## Reduced Balance

Reduced balance is one of the most common factors in knee pain/injury that I see in my clinic, particularly when it comes to individuals over the age of 65. As we hit the 70+ mark there is a reduction in nerve activity, thereby causing reduced balance. As a consequence, older people tend to suffer from falls and knee injuries more readily than their younger counterparts.

Typically, we can lose between 35-40% of our total muscle mass between the ages of 30 and 80; thigh muscles, in particular, weaken faster than others. Hence, the knee joint's functionality is affected and, resultantly, daily activities suffer from poor form.

Ultimately, this means that exercise will cause increased pain and mobility will deteriorate further. In fact, it is not uncommon for the hip extension – which means the ability to move your leg backwards – to reduce by 20% from the age of 75 onward. All these factors greatly contribute to the risk of injury, and as such it is vital that you contact a physiotherapist to correct poor form, strengthen your muscles, and increase your mobility.

Addressing the above will greatly minimise the risk of knee injury and help you live an active lifestyle. For more information about how to self-management tips, as well as for a guide to staying active, I recommend you download my knee guide, here: https://t4physio.co.uk/free-advice-sheets-downloads/knee-pain-advice-sheet/.

## An Accident or Traumatic Fall

It is not unusual to suffer knee pain if you fall and land on your knees, or if you're involved in a traumatic accident such as a road traffic accident. When it comes to knee injuries such as these, you might have swelling, bruising, and stiffness at the back of the knee which affects your walking pattern. You may even hear a minor clicking sound yet experience no major pain.

Despite the seeming lack of pain, however, it is vital that you reach out to a physiotherapist to ensure that there is nothing serious going on. Pain can rear its ugly head later on. A physiotherapist can make sure that your knee is not giving way, that it isn't painfully twisting when the foot it set down, and that it isn't popping, locking, or clicking with pain. Please do not ignore the signs.

The risk of falls increases as we age, therefore it is vital to work on your balance now in order to allow the balance receptors in the knee to stay strong. Balance exercise, Thai-Chi, Yoga/Pilates, and general exercises are excellent to make sure you age well and reduce the risk of falls, particularly if you're aged 75 and over. Normal daily activities such as DIY, gardening, carrying shopping, and cleaning ensures that your lower leg muscles stay strong and that you minimise the risk of weak muscles and joints.

Remember, if you have a knee injury that results in swelling then you should MICE it. This is what the acronym stands for:

M – Movement

In order to avoid muscles weakness, it is important to complete gentle exercises to prevent reduced exercise tolerance.

I – Ice

Apply ice in order to reduce swelling and pain signals to the brain. The ice temporally hinders the pain signals to the brain, hence the pain reduces for about 20-30 minutes with ice application.

C- Compression

If you have ever stayed in hospital for an operation or had a long flight, then you might be familiar with compression stockings. These rather unattractive garments help minimise blood pooling and reduce the risk of developing medical conditions such as Deep Vein Thrombosis, that is, blood clots. So, though unattractive, they are incredibly important.

E- Elevation

It is important to elevate the knee so as to reduce swelling and bruising by encouraging the blood to return to the heart.

So, there you have it: the most common causes for knee pain and, I hope, a deeper understanding of how to mitigate the risks associated with them. Please take head of the advice in this chapter, and if you have any concerns simply reach out to me at **https://t4physio.co.uk/free-advice-sheets-downloads/knee-pain-advice-sheet** or seek medical attention from your local GP.

Let's now move on to the upper section of the leg: the hip and pelvis. Ready? Let's go!

# Chapter 3

## The Hips Don't Lie: Discover the Importance of Your Hips/Pelvis

As I write this, I have just celebrated becoming a father. My amazing wife gave birth to our beautiful baby girl, Talia-Rose – she's instantly become my little princess. What better time than now, then, to chat about the importance of hip and pelvis health?

You may not know this, but the hips/pelvis play an important role when it comes to stability, strength, and overall health. Additionally, if you are a woman then, of course, this area feeds directly into the potential for child bearing. As important as this area is, it can also cause a lot of pain if not treated with care and in a healthful way.

Without going into too many boring scientific details, I would like to talk about some of the issues I typically see in my clinic when it comes treating the hip/pelvis. Why? Because the more you know, the more likely you'll be able to avoid those same mistakes. Come along with me in this very interesting chapter and let's see what so many physiotherapists seem to avoid… the hips/pelvis. Before we jump in, I'd like to make clear that I am not a women's health specialist, but that I none-the-less want to touch on some of the issues related to the hips/pelvis areas so that you can make more informed choices about your own lifestyle choices.

The hip/pelvis joint is the largest ball and socket joint in the body. This might mean nothing to you as you read this, but the truth is that this joint's structure enables us to move unlike any other animal on earth.  It also gives us stability. Anatomically speaking, it is formed by the longer bone of the thigh called the femur, which sits in the socket of the pelvis, namely, the acetabulum. Knowing that it performs all of these vital roles in the body, it's easy to see why an injury in this area could well debilitate you.

When it comes to pain here, then, I'm afraid childbirth can have a lot to do with that. One of the major roles of the hip/pelvis is related to weight bearing. It is not unusual for women to have wider hips than men: this is advantageous during childbearing and for holding toddlers at the hips. When it comes to giving birth like my wife has recently done, women go through a lot of physiological, psychological, and emotional adaptations that result in hip/pelvis discomfort after giving birth. One of the most common pregnancy related issues we find at my clinic is Pelvic Girdle Pain or (PGP). This is simply pain around the pelvis which can be caused by many factors such as previous lower back pain, pelvis pain, hypermobility, or trauma to the pelvis. Due to hormonal changes and pelvis/hip changes during and post-pregnancy, is it not uncommon for some women to suffer with leg length discrepancy, too, whereby one leg becomes slightly shorter than the other leg.

Let's stop and talk about that strange phenomenon whereby one of your legs seem shorter than the other for a minute. Have you ever walked out of the shower and stood in the mirror only to notice that one of your legs was slightly shorter than the other leg? Maybe you tend to stand and lean on one leg more whilst bending the other to feel more balanced?

If the answer is yes to either question, then you're not alone: approximately 60% of the United Kingdom's population will have some sort of leg length discrepancy. This is more common in women than in men, mind you, but it can affect both genders none-the-less. You might very well be wondering what to do if one of your legs seem shorter. I don't blame you!

The thing is, everything in your bloody is linked. Where you see a shorter leg, I may well see some sort of balance discrepancy in the pelvis. You see, your hip/pelvis may alter slightly either due to pregnancy or previous trauma such as a car accident. As a result, this can cause muscle imbalances around the hip/pelvis, back, and legs, thereby resulting in nagging pain/discomfort in different parts of the body. Or, indeed, a trick whereby one of your legs is shorter than the other!

When it comes to treating the hip/pelvis – or the body in general, really – it's less about what you see initially and more about playing the role of detective. The key is finding the root cause of the problem so as to address its oftentimes mysterious side-effects, some of which can be found miles away from the source. A headache that affects the foot? Maybe. Please know, though, that practicing good posture is an incredibly affective way of mitigating the risk of injury. It is astonishing to me that people are not always aware of the role good posture plays in physical health. To underscore this, I'd like to chat about some real-life scenarios and examples of how focussing on daily activities and posture may very well lead you to the root cause of the problem and, consequently, the eradication of pain, specifically in the hip/pelvis area.

# Case Study 1:

A patient attends the clinic with hip/pelvis pain for 4 weeks after giving birth 12-months ago. The patient reports pain of the left side only, especially when socialising with her 12-month old baby. After asking the mother more run-of-the-mill questions, it came to my attention that she is still breast feeding the 12-month year old and always prepares feeding the baby on the right-side breast. This means she is constantly leaning and shortening her left side hip muscles. She prefers carrying the baby on the left hip, and now that she has returned to university she is always carrying her heavy university books on the right shoulder, thereby shortening her left side as she hitches her right shoulder up to prevent the books from slipping.

When she sits down at the computer or to watch TV, she sits crossed legged with her right leg underneath her left buttocks. When she drives, her left armrest is slightly lower than the right thus she has to lean more on her left side when she drives. When she stands in long supermarket queues, she notices that she stands with more weight on her left leg and that she bends her right leg slightly. She finds it strange that, when lying in bed with her legs bent, her left knee appears to be slightly lower than her right knee.

Quite interesting, isn't it? It's clear to see that her normal execution of daily activities appears to be causing her hip pain. In fact, her poor technique and form are actively contributing to her pain/discomfort.

Even if she goes to the best acupuncture session, ultrasound treatment, shockwave therapy, or massage, nothing will help. Why? Because the underlying, root cause of the problem isn't being addressed. She will remain in pain until it is identified and treated correctly. A holistic approach to treating this patient is necessary not only to ease her pain, but to educate her so that she can make informed decisions about her own health and lifestyle and so that she can become an expert in managing her own hip pain.

As we have now briefly addressed the overall physiological issues that can affect the hip/pelvis, let's turn to the muscles around the hip/pelvis, that is, the core muscles. The core muscles are more complex: they can be found deep inside the trunk of the body, and no, they are not just the "six pack" that most people think of. There is a lot more to the core muscles, and in fact, they contribute greatly to correctly posture and, consequently, overall health and a pain free life.

I'll tell you a little secret: I treat many patients with 'six packs', yet so many of them still have poor core muscle strength in their pelvis. Strange, right? Well, no, not really.. You see, there is a difference in the function and role of the superficial muscles – like the six pack – and that of the deep core muscles – like the pelvic floor muscles inside the pelvis.

Let me explain. Without going into too much detail, the 'six pack' muscles usually refer to the superficial muscles found at the front and side of the stomach, whereas the pelvic floor muscles are more complex and lie underneath the trunk. They attach to the spine, thereby allowing us much of our stability in relation to all movement. As a side note, then, if you suffer from lower back pain, it may well be connected to weak pelvic muscles, for instance.

Key pelvic core muscles overlooked by most therapists are the diaphragm muscles known as the 'singing muscles'. These muscles are predominately below the belly button, inside the pelvis, and around the stomach. They give stability to the spine and act as a good base of support during one extreme movement (or not) to the next. They play an important role when it comes to stabilising the hip/pelvis in order to allow for pain free movement of the torso. I advise my patients to check whether they have strong diaphragm muscles by asking them to blow-up a balloon... using the diaphragm, not the face muscles. This exercise certainly looks easier than it is, I promise. Go on, give it a go and see if you can manage it.

The core muscles are really very important when it comes to balance – they are known as the 'pillar' muscles, as they absorb much of the forces from the extremities of the body in order to stabilise you in your activities. As we age, then, it is important it to maintain balance by exercising the core muscles in order to reduce the risk of falls. I see the devastating effects falls can have on a daily basis in my clinic. Hip replacements, shoulder replacements, and knee replacements are but a few of the effects of these types of accidents, particularly for people aged 75 and over.

When it comes to the hip, taking care of your core muscles – and strengthening them – cannot be understated. As I mentioned earlier, the hip joint is made out of the pelvis and the long thigh bone known as the femur. At the top end of the joint we find the femur head; this sits in the round space of the pelvis. Just below the head of the femur is the neck – it looks almost exactly like the structure of your actual neck.

The problem with the neck of the femur is that it has a reduced blood supply which means it takes longer to heal. And that's a real problem as we age. Moreover, when we reach our late 70's, the blood supply is further reduced and the neck of femur becomes weaker. And that's exactly why so many older people suffer hip injuries and, of course, why their recovery times are so much longer. Injury to the hip, particularly the neck of the femur, can result in major surgery/hip replacement and can ultimately reduce quality of life. So, it's clear then that prevention is your best option. As much as hip replacement materials and methods are constantly enhanced, it is so much better to minimise the risk of wear and tear by strengthening your core muscles and practicing good posture. At the end of the day, this will help you mitigate the risk of a fall and, therefore, months in a hospital bed or worse! Having said that, let's talk about practical ways in which you can start making progress when it comes to strengthening those core muscles.

## Pilates/Yoga Exercises

If you've ever completed a Yoga/Pilates session, or experienced a one-to-one gym session with a personal trainer, then you might have heard the words "activate your core". What on the earth does this mean, though? Well, we'll get to that is due course, but let me first distinguish between Pilates and Yoga. Pilates is more core based and uses special equipment to improve your physical strength, flexibility, posture, and mental awareness.

Alternately, Yoga has two parts to it: the health and relaxation elements, and the spiritual/meditation ones. None-the-less, Yoga uses specific body postures to improve flexibility and physical strength, too. Both Pilates and Yoga can make all the difference in your journey to a pain free life, especially when we look at pelvic and hip health. Don't know where to go? Well, at my clinic we offer online and group Pilates and Yoga sessions, so feel free to visit our website and to get in touch for more information: www.t4physio.co.uk

## Bowel Dysfunction

Before we move on to the next section of this chapter, I feel as though it's important to highlight this oftentimes awkward topic when it comes to pelvic muscle strength. Both women and men with weak pelvic core muscles can suffer from weakened bladder and bowel control. In this respect, these same individuals may also experience sexual dysfunction and other health issues. Just as a side note, please know that there is nothing to be ashamed of if you do suffer from these symptoms – there is hope. I encourage to reach out to our team for support, advice, and treatment.

## Tailored Orthotics/Insoles

We now return to leg length discrepancy. As our first case study noted, weakened pelvic muscles may result in pain post-pregnancy or otherwise. In this next case study – during which I prescribed bespoke orthotics to a patient – we look specifically at how imbalanced pelvic and hip muscles can lead to numerous pitfalls down the line.

More so, though, we look at what can be done to mitigate the consequences of this. Take a look:

# Case study 2:

David is 47. He's usually fit and healthy, but has recently pushed himself and has been training for a charity fun run; he has been aiming to reach around 12 miles. A painful hip flare-up began to bother him, so he purchased a pair of 'insoles' to see if running became more comfortable. In doing this, though, he has actually aggravated the problem! He previously visited a podiatrist and was told his right leg was slightly shorter than the left leg and that he therefore needed orthotics. The podiatrist didn't advise how long he would need to use them for nor where to get them from. David asked the podiatrist if he needed to do any exercises, to which the podiatrist responded that he should see a qualified physiotherapist for more information. So, David visited not one, but two physiotherapist clinics before he visited mine: T4 Physio. He wanted to improve his function and running form in preparation for his charity event. Visiting T4 Physio was his last attempt at trying to resolve his ongoing hip pain. At T4, thankfully, David was able to find the root cause of his hip pain via his physiotherapist's three- pronged approach:

1.    Direct therapy of the knee and surrounding muscles.
2.    Shockwave therapy.
3.    Supporting and strengthening exercises.

*An added prescription of bespoke orthotics alongside a bespoke home exercise program and leaflet explaining the benefits of orthotics.

Without the final piece of the puzzle, David's pain would have been ongoing.

Can you see what the difference is between how the physiotherapist handled David's case and how the podiatrist did? It is not enough to prescribe something – you have to be given the tools to enable the treatment to succeed. David had to know how to use the orthotics, why they are essential, and what the parameters for them are. And guess what? Once he knew that, David was well on his way to correcting the imbalance and eradicating his pain.

So, to give you as much information as possible, and therefore the best chance of orthotics working for you, here's the lowdown on orthotics: an orthotic, or insole, is a prescribed medical, removable piece of material that usually goes inside the shoe to correct biomechanics – more on this in chapter 6 – or foot issues, specifically those related to walking or running. Getting the right fit, therefore, is essential. You have to have orthotics that work for you, specifically – generic knock-offs just won't cut it.

It may be that you've tried orthotic/insoles in the past, but were very disappointed. The pain hadn't disappeared and you had presumably spent a considerable amount of money on them, right? Well, you are not alone. In fact, many people feel the same way. Like most things in life, when you know better you do better. On that note, let me explain why your previous orthotics might not have worked.

Firstly, you need to visit a qualified clinician with plenty of experience prescribing orthotics, as not all podiatrists and physiotherapists have the extra training to prescribe them successfully.
If you order online, however, then you need to make sure that the orthotics/insoles are bespoke to fit your unique arches. Secondly, if you do have any significant limb discrepancy, make sure, too, that this is factored in when prescribed orthotic/insoles.

Lastly, and most importantly, you need a tailored rehabilitation exercise program to address the muscle imbalances that might be present in your unique situation so as to complement the orthotics. This is incredibly important. A follow-up exercise program accentuates the effectiveness of the orthotic much, much more than the device itself. And that's precisely why approaching a qualified physiotherapist is so important.

Why then does a well-prescribed, suitable orthotic work so well? The bottom line is that they are tailor made to suit YOU. As mentioned, one size doesn't fit all. In fact, when it comes to orthotics/insoles the difference in feet is incredibly important. An orthotic/insole has to be bespoke so as to give adequate support and to improve gait. Hip/lower back pain, shin splints, and plantar fasciitis are but some of the many medical conditions that can be improved.

How? Well, orthotics can improve your balance by increasing your surface area when you walk or run. Moreover, they address leg length differences in order to reduce pain when you walk or run. Ultimately, they restore normal function and a pain free life.

Before you let go of this book and speed out of the door to get your hands – or feet – on some orthotics, hold your horses. Keep reading.
Orthotics work in conjunction with a holistic approach. They might well be the things that make a difference in your life – getting you back to the things you love to do such as walking your dog or socialising with your children – but please remember that they form part of a holistic, healthy healing plan: a lifestyle that promotes health and mobility above all else.

If you are interested how orthotics might help you, are tired of living with debilitating hip pain, or simply want advice on how to stave off the possibility of future injury, then I invite you to contact us, today. We'd like to offer you a FREE consultation during which you can get a taste of your very own bespoke orthotic/insole using the latest 3D Foot Scanner Technology. To take advantage of this offer, and to make a great decision for your health, simply visit www.t4physio.co.uk/podiatry now.

In closing, I hope this chapter has kick-started your journey to becoming a patient expert, that is, an informed, empowered individual, specifically when it comes to self-managing your hip/pelvic pain. So, now that we've delved into the function of the hip/pelvis and how to self-manage pain in that area, it's time to move up the torso into the back. Aha! It's what you've been waiting for, right? Ready? Let's go!

# Chapter 4
# You Only Have One Back

I have always wondered why people say you only have one back... isn't it obvious? Did I perhaps miss something? Well, I thought so right up until I studied human biology. During my studies I learnt that yes... you do in fact have only one back... and yes, you really, really, REALLY ought to take care of it.

Serious injury to that one back of yours can lead to multiple heart-breaking situations, not least of which is paralysis. I don't really want to start this chapter on a negative note, nor do I want to sound pessimistic, but I do want to stress that this is probably one of the most important chapters in this entire book – YOU ONLY HAVE ONE BACK. In the following pages, you will find vital information that could be nothing short of lifesaving, really.

You see, the back gives you posture, makes you stand nice and tall, gives your body strength, and allows you to strut your stuff out on the street. But even more than your ability to wear a Levi jacket well, your back contains one of the most essential parts of your physical body: the spinal cord.

In essence, the spinal cord is a very big nerve that runs from the back of the brain to your tail bone – and as un-glamorous as that sounds, it's important information to take note of. Why? Well, any injury to the spinal cord can be catastrophic, sometimes even resulting in serious debilitation or worse.
So, pay close attention in this chapter, place a good supporting cushion behind your back as you turn the pages, and let me help you minimise the risk of developing a back injury in the future.

In this chapter I am going to focus on three types of back injury: traumatic back injury, the role of core muscles to support the lower back, and stress/anxiety related back pain. And if you think the latter is a myth, you'd be quite wrong... it is possible to suffer with back pain due chemical imbalances related to stress and anxiety. Stay with me and I will explain exactly how this all works a bit later in this chapter. I will also cover the "red flags" you need to look out for in the medical, but if all this sounds a little bit too much at the moment, not to worry. We'll get to that and much more during the next few pages. Let's get started.

First, we need to take a little look at the anatomy of the back – how can we possibly know how/where/when injury strikes if we don't know much about what the back looks like?

The back is divided into two sections. Initially, we find the upper back, consisting of the thoracic vertebrae bones – 12 in total – and the 7 vertebrae bones of the cervical spine. Then, the lower back section consists of 5 lumbar vertebrae bones. Running between all these vertebrae is the spinal cord. It attaches to the brain to form what is called the central nervous system (CNS). If we think of this entire system as that of a computer, the brain and spinal cord comprise the hard drive of a computer, thereby storing every file on the system.

The CNS controls very important functions like walking and bladder/bowel control, so the body needs it to be "switched on" and functioning at all times. A functioning central nervous system forms the back bone of a healthy, mobile body – and yes, I did intend that pun!

Now, if the spinal cord were involved in a traumatic injury such as serious car accident, it could very well be significantly injured, even despite the protection derived from the surrounding vertebrate, muscles, ligaments, and fascia. Fascia is the thin, transparent membrane that usually sits on top of the muscles covered in nerve endings. Taking care of your back is absolutely essential.

I am not going to spend too long on traumatic lower back injury as most patients we treat at T4 Physio tend to have more non traumatic or gradual onset of lower back pain. I would like to mention the major signs for you to signal for immediate medical attention these flags are well known as the "red flags" in the medical field. These major and most obvious red flags include severe or progressive pins/needless, sharp shooting pain, numbness, reduced sensation in the legs such as major body weakness. Blood and bowel irritation, Sensory loss to the gentle area and unexplained weight loss.

Please remember that, if you or a loved one suffer with any of the above, don't try to self-manage the pain or discomfort. It's extremely important that you seek medical advice, treatment, and guidance to prevent serious injury further down the line. Let me tell you about my own back injury story – I think this is an important story to share because I really want you to start thinking of your back as one of your most important assets. My experience as a patient taught me a lot about how I can best help those who seek treatment in my clinic, and I hope I can help you, too.

Being a physio, I never thought I would suffer with back pain. And let me tell you a little secret, the same is true for most clinicians… until it happens to them! I was 28 and hadn't had a care in the world – I had that naïve belief that I was immortal in the way only a 20-something can. How wrong I was!

When I initially qualified as physio my first job involved telephone consultation physio - this meant I had limited standing time during which to give hands-on treatment. Instead, it involved prolonged sitting at a desk and completing telephone physiotherapy. If you knew me then you'd understand that this entire situation was less than ideal for me – I'm a very active person and enjoy moving around.

So, in a nutshell it felt like a customer service job – not only was I not really healing people the way in which I wanted to, but I felt somewhat tethered to a desk. I would spend 5-6 hours a day on the phone, giving health advice and exercise programs to patients. Sure, it was excellent for my bank balance, but for my body... well that's a different matter. My back was literally cracking at the end of my working day. I could hear it!

It was only a matter of time before I found myself overwhelmed by the most excruciating, stabbing pain across my lower back. It literally felt like somebody walked up behind me with a sharp knife and stabbed me in the spine. It took all the air out of my lungs and – I'm not ashamed to admit it – all the bravery I had. I was incredibly frightened to take a breath. And you know what the most frustrating this was? It simply came out of nowhere – I didn't pick anything up, I wasn't in an accident, and I hadn't fallen.

Well, that's what I thought for a few moments until my physio-brain kicked in: I had suddenly experience the culminating effects of chronic back pain with sciatica nerve irritation caused by my 2 years of working a sedentary physio job. And I woke up to the fact that... yes... I, too, only have one back! I soon learnt that pain does not respect a person or care if you're in the medical field or not...pain is pain, and it's awful to experience. And now... I'm here writing this book because I never want you to feel this way.

As we move ahead, we'll now dive into those three different types of pain I mentioned right at the beginning of this chapter. As we move through the three categories, keep a look out for signs of your own back pain so that you can gain the information best suited to helping you find relief from your discomfort.

# Back Pain that Creeps Up on You

Now let's move on and talk about back pain that gradual sneaks up on you without warming, this is what I call the "silent back pain". Sure, this type of back injury may not initially seem as serious as a trauma induced one but it certainly cannot be understated as it can be debilitating.

Taking action, here, may well mean the difference between a life filled with ongoing dull ache back pain, or one filled with activity and mobility.

The silent back pain or non-traumatic back pain injuries are also known as know "chronic injuries" as they generally occur over a prolonged period of time. Their lengthy development is due to multiple factors working, of which some include posture, manual handling techniques, and repetitive movements to name but a few.

Many times, I see patients come into the clinic with excruciating, daily back pain. This isn't all that surprising given the prevalence of back pain in an ever more sedentary population, I'm afraid, but it is still concerning. I ask my patients to think of the "trigger" for the pain, and whilst most if not all reference picking up the bin, brushing their teeth, or doing the washing, it is never quite as it seems. You see, the onset of pain doesn't necessary indicate the cause of the pain.

Yes, that' right. What if poor posture spanning over the last 5 years finally cause your back to give in when you picked the bin up this morning? What if the way in which you've tied your shoes over your lifetime finally caused your back to say "nope, no more"? What if your back simply couldn't take the strain of months of imbalance? Well, something has got to give!

Habits, posture, and balance matter! Yes, it can sometimes be difficult to think back to all the bad habits accumulated over your lifetime, but if you don't… you'll never know why that darn bin caused you all this back trouble in the first place! And that's precisely why I can this type of injury the "silent injury". You have to find its voice.

## Where else could my back pain be coming from?

It is important to stress that lower back pain is complex to treat and there're several multifactorial causes that are physical and non-physical like stress and anxiety.

One of the common physical elements that can contribute to lower back pain includes a weak core and pelvic floor muscles. Yes that's right! Before you start to panic, please let me explain.

The weak core gets the blame for most aches and pains in the body and although it can contribute to lower back it must not be isolated as the only cause. Even though the stomach, abdominal and pelvic floor muscles are at the front of the body, weakness in these muscles can encourage a forward lean posture also known as lordotic posture which in turn can irritate the lower back. The reason is back muscles work in unison with the stomach muscles to allow the spine to move in different directions and the core muscles act as an anchor to stabilise the trunk to allow spinal movement and prevents it from being flimsy.

# Pregnancy

It was a privilege to witness my wife Bernadette give birth to our little girl Talia-Rose and I certainly respect women far more after observing all the minor and major changes throughout her pregnancy.

Pregnancy related lower back is common during pregnancy, when giving birth and postpartum. Needless to say, weight gain during a healthy pregnancy is invertible which means the spine has to support the extra weight to minimise lower back as the uterus expands to accommodate the baby.

As well hormonal and posture changes muscles separation of the abdominal muscles due to uterus expansion can result in lower back pain. During either natural or C-Section the core muscles can suffer trauma as the baby is being delivered and this can cause lower back pain during the delivery and postpartum period too. If the core and pelvic floor muscles are never rehabbed or strengthened postpartum then conditions such as pelvic girdle pain (PGP) can be experienced by some women.

Although PGP symptoms are typically reported at the front of the pelvis it can also cause uncomfortable symptoms due to misalignment of the pelvis caused by pelvic rotation due to hormonal changes which can result in sacroiliac joint dysfunction (SIJ) pain at the bottom of the back and functional leg length discrepancy. Yes, I know! Pregnancy can really mess up the body so let me explain what pregnancy related functional leg length discrepancy is and how it can cause lower back pain. Due to the pelvic rotation and separation triggered by hormones during birth misalignment of the pelvis can result in one side of the pelvis slightly elevated and appear as if one leg is shorter than the other one. As a result the spine can be out of alignment and contribute to poor posture and back pain.

The truth is, differences in leg length could be contributing to the back pain and poor posture, Yes, that' right! Before you start to panic this can treated with bespoke orthotics/insoles given alongside a bespoke exercise program. Please note pregnancy is not only of the potential causes of leg length differences, if you constantly sit on your wallet or on one other leg or with your legs crossed then this can potentially cause back pain.

The can encourage muscle imbalance as the pelvis can tilt to one side and can consequently cause hip hitching thereby resulting in a slight lifting. And thus functional leg length discrepancy can be born... affecting the feet, knee, hip/back, and in some cases even the neck/shoulder.

Here is personal story from my wife Bernadette experienced post giving birth to our daughter Talia-Rose. This story is encourage you to seek medical advice if you're suffering from the same symptoms even years postpartum.

My name is Bernadette Dangarembizi and before being discharged home from the hospital one of the women's health physios came to tell me about the importance of pelvic floor exercises. I was handed a piece of paper with a website address for demo videos.

Unfortunately once I got home and tried to access the website my computer said 'url not found' simply put the computer said no.

I became busy with mummy duties until I noticed I was having the urge to pee more often.... I recalled the need for pelvic floor exercises and decided to check out some videos on YouTube in search for decent Kegel exercises.

I have always been hopeless at DIY and there were way too many videos to choose from.... I will sum it up as a sea of confusion.

My post pregnancy aches have been the gift that kept on giving... As the weeks progressed I noticed I was getting pain in my ankles and the bottom of my feet. I initially put it down to being on my feet most of the day..... The problem didn't go away and I started taking paracetamol at bedtime.

I called my GP as I was now having back pain and wrist pain shooting into my shoulder. He recommended taking an anti-inflammatory i.e. Ibuprofen. I did not want to continue taking pain killers as I was not keen on taking dealing with the symptoms.

I eventually booked in an assessment session at T4 Physio clinic and it's the best thing I ever did. My core was in a mess, I had developed poor posture and I found out that the pelvic exercises I had been doing were outdated. I am having ongoing maintenance sessions and no longer need pain killers, phew!

*Perhaps you are like me, a new mum or working from home and struggling with back pain, wrist pain from repetitive tasks. Consider booking in for an assessment, a good chat with the lovely Team at T4 Physio and a chance to say goodbye to pain killers that you are relying on.*

Your body is incredibly interconnected, and this is why my team and I use a holistic detailed assessment approach as part of our patient-centered treatments. Everything connects – and if you don't look at the body as a whole then you'll never figure out the root cause. So, an understanding of the body as a whole is imperative, no matter who you turn to for help.

Let me wrap up this section with my top 5 self-management tips before I talk about stress and anxiety. These tips will give you some of the tools you need to manage your back pain or other minor injuries particularly if you have no other underlying medical issues.

1.      It is important to remain active and to continue with modified daily activities as much as possible. The worst thing you can do is to remain inactive as this can increase back pain and reduce muscle strength, flexibility and exercise tolerance.

2.      Try to alter your position regularly every 30 minutes in order to make sure you do not compromise on your posture. Believe it or not, you are actually better off lying on your back on a flat surface than sitting on a chair. Why? Well, sitting for prolonged periods can increase the pressure across your back, cause discomfort, and prolong the healing process.

3.     Medication should be used not to mask the pain, but to manage the pain. It should be used to reduce the pain in order to complete exercises or a rehab program. Examples of pain medication may include anti-inflammatories and paracetamol, though much more addictive variants, are available – please be aware of the medication you take, as not all of them are created equal.

4.     Heat/ice therapy is another great traditional home remedy you can use to manage symptoms naturally. This form of treatment can be used on its own or as one combined with other treatments. Both ice/heat can help to eliminate pain, spasms and swelling.

Gentle exercises will minimise stiffness and swelling while promoting independence and mobility . This is incredibly important for maintaining muscle strength. When it comes to muscles, well, you either use them or you lose them, I'm afraid.
They need to be used in order to remain healthy and strong and, as a consequence, to provide adequate support for the bones and other tissues in your body. General exercise may include swimming, cycling, and walking. If severe symptoms are not showing any signs of reducing 1-2 weeks later a physiotherapist can provide additional support. During the physiotherapy sessions advice and exercises will be provided, and if this fails other soft tissue techniques such as manipulation, massage, and acupuncture may be useful.

Something to think about: treating your back pain may have to do a lot more with what you've done over a period of time or the trauma caused by pregnancy than it has with what you're doing right now.

Make sure you tell your healthcare provider about any injuries or bad habits you may have, as the clue to your root cause may well be found there. If you would like to book a free 15 minutes consultation to get to the bottom of your back pain then please visit our website: https://t4physio.co.uk/contact/ or email us at info@t4physio.com.

## Can Stress/Anxiety cause Back pain?

Now that I have highlighted some of the main physical reasons why you might suffer with back pain, let me now continue by exploring stress/anxiety related back pain. If you've never considered stress a strong contender for the main culprit causing your back pain, then it's time to open your mind.

When left to their own devices, stress and anxiety can potentially result in oftentimes debilitating back pain. Would I be right in assuming that you're wondering just how that may happen? Well, with more and more research on the subject being produced on a daily basis, it has become increasingly clear that the link between back pain, stress, and anxiety is a lot more impactful that it may first appear to be.

Firstly, let me give you a basic chemistry lecture. No Nash! Well, yes. Chemistry can be fun, right? We have four major hormones that control the body and its stress levels: serotonin, dopamine, oxytocin, and endorphins. I'm sure you've heard of them before.

They function in a very complex chemical balance – tightrope walkers each and every one of them. So, any alteration in the level of one of more of these hormones can result in anxiety/stress and can ultimately cause or exacerbate back pain. This reason is simple and yet so complex, stress even though is a psychological response it can manifest physically and exacerbate back pain.

Here is how stress can negatively impact the body especially if becomes chronic. Pupils delate, heightened senses to hearing can affect sleep and inadequate sleep results in general body fatigue. Stress can release cortisone which is stress-hormone that can cause muscle tension as the body is ready for flight of fight due to release adrenaline hence, we can end up with neck/shoulder tension as a result of stress.

Breathing rate can increase as the muscles use more oxygen and the oxygen rich blood to reach the arms and legs for activity and this can also result in general fatigue as the body tenses due to circulating stress hormones. All these changes can leave us feeling general sick and unwell therefore stress has to be addressed to prevent all the physical changes above that stop us staying active and doing the things we love.

In simple terms, anxiety is triggered when chemicals in the body are not balanced. Serotonin, also known as the "feelings" hormone, controls our bowel movements, sleep, mood, and emotions. This hormone can reduce because of a number of reasons: lack of adequate rest and chronic pain to name but two. Now, over time this psychological distress in the brain can potentially manifest physically, thereby resulting in physical pain/discomfort in the back and other parts of the body.

Similarly, reduced physical activity can also cause psychological distress and even worsen pain in the back and in the body as a whole. Essentially, both the brain and the body are complexly connected and are in constant communication. If one is affected then the other is invariable equally affected, thereby leading to "dis- ease" or disease of the body.

It is vitally therefore important to have personal coping strategies and beliefs in order to self-manage your anxiety and stress so as to avoid catastrophic thinking. Yes, it's about as serious as it sounds. Catastrophic thinking, that is, always thinking of the worst-case scenario, can have a direct effect on the body; it can cause or increase physical pain that was not present before the manifestation.

The other hormone to be aware of is called dopamine. This hormone is responsible for brain activity, emotional control, and attention. You may very well be using some of your dopamine as you're reading this right now! It is worth mentioning that dopamine is highly addictive and if not managed properly it can end up controlling many of your decisions in its favour. It is nonetheless a very important hormone and its levels need to remain stable in order to reduce stress.

Now, imagine if both serotonin and dopamine levels were reduced in the body. This would lead to catastrophic changes within the body all due to that particular chemical imbalance. As a result, you're not only emotionally wrecked – your brain cannot control your distress – but due to a lack of control, fatigue, sadness, and upset, your back has now taken on the stress and anxiety and you have pain! The circle is perpetuated – more pain, more stress, more pain. Something has to be done!

Now, if we factor in pre-existing attitudes, medical conditions, and social factors in too, then you can only imagine how bad your back pain, anxiety, and stress can become. This is known as learnt helplessness. When the pain first occurs, it affects the sensitivity of pain receptors, but then when pain lasts for a long period (2-3 months) it becomes chronic pain… the related brain function focuses on the emotions causing anxiety and stress. And the circle continues.

Another hormone is commonly known as the "love hormone". It is typically released when a mother gives birth to a new-born or when we have sex.
It is known as oxytocin. This hormone is very powerful and it plays a major role in the body, most typically when we have physical contact with others. Happily it also boosts our immune systems! In comparison to dopamine, which is responsible for instant gratification, oxytocin is longer lasting and leave you feeling secure. Another special characteristic of oxytocin is linked to physical wound healing, too. Happiness and healing? Sounds pretty good, right? Well, reduced levels of this hormone – due to stress/anxiety – can also exacerbate your back pain symptoms: as you focus on the pain, and not on things that give you pleasure, things become worse and worse.

Last, but by no mean least, we have endorphins… also known as the "runners' high hormones". These hormones are usually released when we exercise the body beyond our comfort zones in order to improve exercise tolerance and maintain health/fitness. These hormones also help us to fight pain and give us a "high feeling" that can inadvertently reduce body pain. I elaborate how this happens in a later chapter, so stay tuned. When it comes to endorphins, it's important that there are no large dips in their levels, as any fluctuation may well result in more stress, thereby leading to pain.

So, in summary, each of these chemicals play an important role in keeping us not only emotionally stable, but also physically and mentally fit and well. Managing stress is incredibly important, as keeping your hormones stable plays a huge role in preventing and/or healing back pain. Please be sure to introduce wellness regimes into your life – more on this in a later chapter 8.

Back pain can be due to traumatic injuries, non-traumatic injuries, or stress and anxiety. More research is being published daily, but the common denominator in every paper is finding the root cause remains the best way of healing pain permanently and safety. I hope this chapter has given you the information you need to find the answers you seek. For more tips, advice, and hands-on treatment for your back pain, why not give us a call or visit www.t4physio.co.uk or email info@t4physio.com now?

As we head into the next chapter of the book, please take a moment to reflect on your habits, past injuries, and stress levels – true healing comes from a place of knowledge. Now, let us move up the body and into the shoulders and neck. In our 'body part' chapters, so buckle up and let's get going!

# Chapter 5

# Neck/Shoulder Pain: It's a pain in the Neck

If you suffer from neck and/or shoulder pain, then you already know how debilitating it can be. Not only can it steal your joy, but it can severely decrease your mobility and energy levels. You may be asking yourself why you're suffering with the agonising, daily pain related to neck and shoulder issues, but I can assure you that you're not alone and that there is a way out of it.

I have treated many individuals with similar issue and most managed to recover apart from a few exceptions. What's more, most of them lead active, healthy, happy lives now! So, there really is hope.

Most of the patients treated at T4 Physio clinic eventually do admit that they thought the pain would go away with painkillers and without treatment. I think this is a natural response – we all want to believe that things will get better of their own accord. The truth is, though – and my patients will attest to this – is that by waiting and taking medications the pain got worse; they got even more frustrated and lethargic.

Does this sound like you? Maybe you are frustrated or feeling confused – many different doctors, treatments, diagnoses, and out-of-the-box approaches later, and nothing has gotten better. You probably still don't really know what's wrong. With this in mind, this chapter will speak about the most common causes of neck pain and shoulder and how to manage your symptoms, particularly to prevent ongoing chronic pain. Remember, knowledge is power! Let's get straight to it.

As per usual, let's start with a visual. The neck is composed of 7 bones known as vertebrae – these bones make up the cervical spine. Other supporting structures include discs, ligaments, and tendons, all of which work together to make up the neck. The amount of receptors and nerves in the neck is overwhelming – so it really isn't surprising that you may be experiencing pain, here. Everything is connected – from your neck, to your shoulders, and even down into your spine.

The main function of the neck is to support the head and to protect the spinal cord, whilst all the while facilitating movement. In between the vertebrae are discs which act as shock absorbers to absorb impact so as to protect the skeletal structure. The muscles and strong ligaments keep the neck upright and protect the spinal cord at the same time. It's interesting, right?

And all these intricate structure still allow for what is arguably the most dynamic area of your body: the neck is very flexible so as to allow the head to move. And yet, all this precision lays bare the very real potential for serious injury: trauma, overuse, injury, wear and tear, and sudden impacts can all cause problems in neck.

There're many causes of neck injuries, from muscle strain, poor sleep hygiene, whiplash injuries road traffic accidents, and ligaments and vertebrae damage, all the way through to simple careless movement.
On the other hand, neck problems may be due to general wear and tear and underlying conditions such as osteoarthritis. It is worth knowing that while neck pain can be sudden and unexpected, it can also develop slowly, over time, and without.

Neck tension can slowly build up overtime or come on suddenly if the neck muscles are strained resulting in neck stiffness, spasms and tightness. Here are some of the typical causes of neck tension reported by most of the client that visit T4 Physio clinic that you need to be aware of and avoid them to minimise ongoing neck tension.

The most common one is poor posture caused by the head pocking forward and the shoulder rounding forwards results in misalignment of the spine thus causing tension as the neck muscles are forced to work extra hard. Teeth grinding is when you grind or clench your teeth resulting in neck and jaw tension.

Repetitive motion or sustained poor neck posture required in some occupations can also result in neck unwanted neck tension. Last but not least is high stress levels increase neck tension due to release of stress hormone called cortisone which causes involuntary muscle contraction.

At times you might find holding your shoulders up close to your ears due to stress which in turn creates tension and trigger points on top of the shoulders. One of the questions I get asked in the clinic is "Nash, what is a trigger point?". Well, my answer is usually in lay terms and along the lines of, trigger points is sensitive spot found in the muscle tissue that can cause pain to another area of the body known as referred pain.

Typical areas that trigger point like to hide is the neck and although there no clear cause identified, stress and repetitive muscle usage is strongly linked to trigger points. One of the common manifestations of trigger point we see in most patients is development of tension headaches as the nodule of the muscle fiber hardens thus causing a radiation of pain towards the head.

Now, I don't have to be a neurologist surgeon to know that tension headaches are very complex. Migraines are slightly different to headaches in that they occur when you have a headache on one side only – these can be so painful that they can debilitate you for days if you're not careful. Common causes of headaches themselves include stress, neck tension, inadequate sleep, allergies, sinus, and binge drinking alcohol to name but a few.

The one cause that I want to focus on – one that we frequently see at here at T4 Physio – is related to stress. These headaches, known as stress-tension headache, are caused by our reactions to personal issues, money worries, and job stress, for example. All of these worries cause the stress hormone, namely cortisol, to be released.

Now, in some cases the release of cortisol is good, as it increases the blood sugar levels in the bloodstream and improves brain function. All sounds rosy, doesn't it? Well, the downside is that the constant release of cortisol for prolonged periods can cause issues like headaches and a comprised immune system. As such, your stress needs to be mitigates accordingly.

When the body perceives something to be a threat, your nervous system responds by releasing a flood of stress hormones, including both adrenaline and cortisol. Again, this is perfect if you're being chased by a bear, but it is less than ideal if you're watching "Friends" in your armchair at home.

Fight or flight applies to situations that are otherwise unique to our general way of life: UFO landings, snake bites, and a sudden outbreak of rabies. When this response is triggered in frequently experienced situations – driving to school, picking up a pizza, or checking your bank balance – things get complicated. Chronic stress can result in neck tension, thereby triggering headaches which can often leave you debilitated.

Now that we have covered the effects and causes of the neck tension and tension headaches , let's talk about neck tension caused by trauma or accident.

## Whiplash Injury Disorder

As a trained medical expert, I attended extensive medical training to be able to give evidence in court as a physiotherapist expert therefore whiplash syndrome or disorder is the type of injury I am familiar with. Car accidents are usually the common causes of whiplash injuries that I treat and they're normal caused by sudden acceleration or deceleration of the neck, as can be experienced in a road traffic, can wreak absolutely havoc on the neck.

A sudden, unexpected movement and cause serious injury – we can see these type of "whiplash" injuries in car accident victims and older victims who suffered a fall, for example.
Injuries such as these can result in damage to the bones, soft tissue, and ligaments around the neck which, in turn, can set of a chain reaction down the body into the back and hips. Whiplash injury can also affect the back and shoulders, thus it is always advisable to seek medical advice even if you suffer a minor injury. If left untreated it can reduce movement and can eventually lead to long term disability.

As I mentioned before referred pain is when the pain one part of the body that can trigger a problem or pain to another part of the body. In some cases this can indicate some more serious that requires urgent medical attention and in some cases it's more general muscle/joint aches/pain rather than anything sinister.

For example, neck pain that is exacerbated with physical activities may indicate heart problem or if you get constant pins/needles, shooting pain or numbness going down both arms then in this case you require urgent attention. It worth pointing out that it is not uncommon to have referred pain in the hand/fingers, wrist, elbow and shoulders caused by neck tension and nerve irritation in the neck. Don't be surprised if a clinician start to treat your neck in order to alleviate symptoms in your shoulder, elbow, wrist and hands/fingers.

Remember, it's better to be safe than sorry so if in doubt seek medical attention as waiting for it to away could only make it a lot worse.

I'd like to offer you some self-management tips that you can implement right now in order to reduce the pain in your neck and/shoulder.
Avoid sleeping on thick pillows, or more than two pillows, as this can cause one side of the neck to shorten and develop tension. You want to make sure the pillow is not too thick and that it offers enough support for you to sleep comfortably. A memory foam pillow, that is, one which keeps your neck in a natural position, is highly recommended as it would go a long way to minimise neck/shoulder pain. When you have a poor sleep hygiene tension can develop in the neck, thereby resulting in pain.

Minimise poor posture. Desk jobs breed poor posture, so it is important to be aware of how to rectify this. Jobs involving long periods of sitting in front of a computer or a laptop can directly affect your back, shoulders, and neck. Be sure to contact a physiotherapist for advice on sitting and managing these types of environments.

If you carry a bag around for prolonged periods, please make sure you switch the sides on which the bag rests regularly. Do this to minimise the risk of developing shoulder tension. Wearing the bag across the back allows the weight to be distributed evenly and reduces the chances of developing shoulder tension – you may want to consider this option instead.

If you have a job where you are sedentary or desk based for most of the day, then it is important to correct poor sitting habits and to regularly move around as much as possible. To improve posture you can wear a brace so as to ensure your head, neck, and shoulders remain in an optimal position. A posture brace is useful to prevent forward rounding of the neck/shoulders. However, if used continually it can cause weakness in the core muscles.

Reduce stress related neck tension. As mentioned in an earlier chapter, it is almost impossible to avoid stress entirely, but it is certainly worth a shot. Try to manage your stress insofar as possible. If stress is not managed correctly, it can result in physical tension and headaches.

I will wrap up this neck section with the "red flags" symptoms that you need to be on the lookout for, particularly when it comes to seeking medical attention:

- Neck pain moving down into both arm/legs.
- Loss of bowel or bladder control.

- Severe headaches/migraines.
- Numbness, tingling, or weakness in the arms or legs.
- Affected balance or coordination.
- Fever.
- Double vision, blurred speech, swallowing issues, drop attacks, nausea.

Treatment usually involves physiotherapy consisting of specific neck exercises and a tailor-made rehabilitation program designed to restore movement, reduce pain, and increase exercise tolerance.

To download a FREE Neck and Shoulder guide then please visit our website **https://t4physio.co.uk/free-advice-sheets-downloads/neck-and-shoulder-pain-advice-sheet/**.

Other treatment methods such as acupuncture, ultrasound, and heat therapy are known to be effective at reducing pain and improving range of motion and function, though physiotherapy remains the safest and most effective option. Ice therapy may also give you some results, as 5-10 minutes of ice application for up to 5 times a day can go some ways to reducing swelling. For more information about the benefits of physiotherapy treatment please read Chapter 9.

## The Shoulder: One of the Most Painful Joints in the Body

Now, I want to talk about the shoulder. This joint has the potential to be one of the most painful joints in the body. Why? Simply because of the incredible physiology within it. Let me start by explaining the basic structures that make up the shoulder – I'll then share with you some of the common injuries and how to treat them.

The shoulder is a ball and socket joint. This means it has a "ball like socket" as well as synovial fluid to allow for multidirectional movement, Of course, this type of movement is incredibly important when it comes to completing tasks such as washing our hair, playing sports such tennis, and doing many other daily activities. Mexican wave, anyone?

So it is therefore understandable that the shoulder has to be flexible – in order to effective execute the activities you need it to, your shoulder needs to be able to step up to the plate. It also has to be very strong.

As such, it is made up of three bones: the arm bone, the shoulder bone, and the collar bone. All three of these add support and strength with the help of their surrounding soft tissue, ligaments, tendons, and joint capsule. The shoulder joint also contains the brachial plexus nerve – this run into the arm, thereby making it very sensitive to pain if injured. What's more, even though the shoulder blade is at the back of the shoulder, it plays a very important role in stabilising the shoulder as a whole, especially when it comes to moving your arms. Lastly, rotator cuff muscles – four of them – help stabilise the shoulder further.

Let's delve into some of the more common types of injuries you might encounter in the shoulder – remember, my aim is to educate you on the ways in which you may have injured your shoulder… knowledge is power!

Thickening of the tendons known as tendinopathy is a common shoulder injury – this condition can severely restrict movement and cause you to stop doing the activities you love. How does it happen? Well, due to the shoulder joint being a very complex one – with lots of muscles, nerves and tendons crossing each other constantly – it is incredibly interconnected. Thus, it is understandably vulnerable to getting inflamed as a result of an irritation of tendons rubbing on bone or simply being overused.

Think of a cricket player – can you imagine how often he/she uses his/her arm to bowl? How about the muscles he/she activates when he/she reaches overhead and spins the ball towards the batter?
Well, simply imagining the complexity of movement in this example will give you a good idea of why the shoulder can be so easily hurt. Now, you don't need to be a cricket player suffer from a shoulder injury. Shoulder issues can arise following mundane everyday tasks such as cleaning above head height, sweeping the flood, or carrying heavy laundry. Not quite a Shane Ward movement, but still.

The shoulder muscles can be broken into two categories; prime movers and stabilisers. The former are the big muscles around the shoulder – the deltoid and upper traps (prime movers)– and the latter are the smaller muscles inside the shoulder that gives stability to allow range of  shoulder motion  and without pain. The prime movers are the bigger major muscles of the shoulder that we can see on the outside like the deltoids and upper trapezius (shoulder muscles that sit on top of the shoulders).

However, it is important to highlight that in order for these bigger muscles surrounding the shoulder to work properly they require the assistance of the smaller muscles inside the shoulder which are called the big four rotator cuff muscles. Supraspinatus, infraspinatus, Subscapularis and Teres Minor are the names of the rotator cuff muscles for those that are interested in knowing the names. These rotator cuff muscles play a vital role to allow smooth and pain-free shoulder movement across all 4 shoulder joints when they're functioning correctly.

I will not turn this into a anatomy lecture but I do want to highlight that mundane daily task like poor posture, repetitive shoulder/arm movements, poor sleep hygiene and regular sporting activities are some of the mundane activities that can contribute to shoulder dysfunction.

I cannot help but notice that more and more people are walking around with their heads buried in the phone, prolonged desk-based sitting reinforced with working from home, increase in stress and anxiety due to the Covid-19 pandemic resulting in shoulder tension and reduced physical activity to only name a few of the contributing factors to shoulder issues.

The rotator cuff tendons that are likely to wear and tear and cause inflammation as the ageing process kicks-in from the age of 40 plus. Due to the busyness of the shoulder joint the rotate cuff muscles help to "rotate" the arm while acting like a "cuff" during movement they become a prime suspect to be impinged as they can rub on the bone or other soft tissue. Hence shoulder impingement injury is very common and if you have experienced shoulder pain before then you know it can be very painful and debilitating with the healing time lasting 3-6 months.

The humble shoulder blade in another crucial landmark of the human anatomy that play crucial role in giving the shoulder the stability it needs to function correctly. The shoulder blade which is a large triangular shaped bone hides behind the back and this is one of the reasons why it's easily missed. It important to note any dysfunction to the rotator cuff muscles or any of the muscle surrounding the shoulder blade can result in restricted and pain movement of the arm especially when completing normal daily activities like gardening, carrying shopping and shopping.

Due to the posterior location of the shoulder blade, it is possible for it to "wing" that means instead of sticking to the ribcage it lifts away from the ribcage creating a gap between the shoulder blade and the ribcage. As a result of this alteration shoulder pain can be birthed usually caused by poor posture of rounded shoulders/neck and shoulder muscles imbalances.

Typically, individuals that present with a winged shoulder blame can potentially have tightness in the chest/pectoral areas too, as the muscles at front of the shoulder become more dominant due to the rounded shoulder and inactive the back muscles. Continued usage and movement of a dysfunctional shoulder can then start to create more tension and shoulder pain which further debilitates the shoulder. If left untreated these tension spots can increase in size and restricted movement and trigger more shoulder pain that can eventually travel down the arm and fingers and cause referred pain. "Referred pain", meaning the pain originates in a place removed from where the pain is now. If this is the case for you, then appropriate physiotherapy treatment will be able to reduce your symptoms and help you get back to the happy, mobile, pain free life you deserve.

# Stress Related Shoulder Tension

It is important to be aware that shoulder tension and stiffness can be secondary due ongoing stress and anxiety. You see when we are stressed something else other than pulling our hair is happening beneath the surface that we might not be aware of.

Hormones are being released and one of these hormones being released is known as cortisol which is a stress hormone that can work in our favour or not. The positive effect of cortisol is it increases the blood sugar levels in the bloodstream and improves body and brain function to allow the body to be equipped to take action, fight or flight response.

However, the constant release of cortisol means the body is in a constant state to fight/fight mood and this is not good at all. If this continues to happen regularly for prolonged periods then general fatigue/feel exhausted, tension headaches and shoulder tightness/pain can start to manifest. Think for a moment. have you ever walked around with your shoulders hunched up for a while (hopefully you're not doing it now as you read this book) or had a stressful day resulting is slow elevation of your shoulders to your ears as the tension intensifies?

Well, this is the negative effect of cortisol taking its toll on your body, and if left untreated it can quickly develop tension spots resulting in further tension and stiffness. You don't have oto suffer in silence so keep reading this chapter to get the solution for you or a loved one.

# What is Frozen About my Shoulder?

To understand what frozen shoulder is, we first need to understand that between the ball and socket of the shoulder joint there is a sack of fluid called the synovial fluid. This fluid allows the shoulder to move more easily.

It is not uncommon to see that, between the ages of 40 and 60, the shoulder joint can stiffen as the synovial fluid thickens, thereby resulting in restricted movement in the shoulder. And suddenly you have frozen shoulder!

The early onset of frozen shoulder can be triggered by many factors such as Rotator cuff repair, shoulder surgery, and wear and tear of the shoulder joint or early onset of arthritis are also known to trigger frozen shoulder, too. However, I would advise against diagnosing yourself! You still need to undergo physiotherapy tests, and potentially and MRI or X-Ray to ascertain the real cause of your immobility in the shoulder.

The good news about frozen shoulder, however, is that it has been known to resolve itself within 3 years in most cases. However, this is not always the case. There are normally 3 stages present in an individual's frozen shoulder journey: the freezing stage, whereby the individual reports pain with limited range of motion – this tends to be the early onset stage, that is, before it progresses; the frozen stage, whereby pain can disappear yet shoulder stiffness and tightness remain albeit with significantly reduced range of motion; the thawing stage, whereby the shoulder's mobility begins to return with minimal pain.

What can we do to you or a loved one? If you or a loved one is suffering with shoulder pain or restricted shoulder movement then put a stop to it today. Here T4 physio we have offer physiotherapy solutions that can reduce pain and improve your exercises tolerance.

These solutions include acupuncture, shockwave therapy, ultrasound, and heat/ice therapy, exercises and to name a few (Read Chapter 9 to find more details about the benefits of these physiotherapy treatments).

If you would like to find more resources and self-management tips for shoulder pain then visit our website to https://t4physio.co.uk/free-advice-sheets-downloads/neck-and-shoulder-pain-advice-sheet/ to download a free guide sheet. If you wish to go straight to the treatment table or book a FREE 15 mins consultation with a shoulder expect then please don't hesitate to contact us on info@t4phyiso.com or visit our website www.t4physio.co.uk.

As we move into the next part of the book we're taking a deeper look at exercise followed by diet in the chapter after that. We're into the nitty gritty of making a change in your life, and I hope you'll join me as we turn the corner towards a healthier, happier, pain-free you!

# Chapter 6
# The Importance of Exercise

We've moved through the parts of the body as they relate to health and a pain free lifestyle. It's now time to turn to the body as a whole, that is, how all its composite parts work in unison to help us live the best, healthiest lives we can. Of course, as with many things in life, health really is a choice, and in a world where we are bombarded with bad food choice, sedentary activities, and generally unhealthy behaviours on a daily basis, that choice can be really hard. I'm here to help though. So if you're ready to get started on a healthful journey, let's take that first step together. And guess what? That first step is really the beginning of movement… yup, you guessed it… this chapter is all about the importance of exercise both in a pain free lifestyle as well as in a life filled with health, longevity and happiness. Let's get moving!

So, what does it actually mean to exercise, why is it important, and what is the daily recommend duration and type of exercise? These are complex questions, and I'm afraid to say… they don't have simple answers.

Each individual will have different requirements, but the main thing is that, no matter what you do, you have to remember to move! As you know by now, movement is the key to a pain free life – the more you move, the more your muscles and joints are lubricated, and the better chance you have of avoiding injury, maintaining a healthy weight, staving off illness, and being generally more content in life. It's a win-win.

And hey… movement isn't simply about running for an hour on the treadmill. It's about dancing while you clean, getting off the bus a stop early, ditching the car and taking your bike, or running around the garden with your kids. The window of opportunity for exercise is there, you just have to find it.

Let's get back to basics. As a general definition, exercise is an activity that requires physical effort sustain or improve health and fitness. But really, exercise just means that you're physically moving. You're moving your body to get your heart rate up a little. Why? Well, as humans we are designed to use our muscles, or ultimately, to lose them. As we age, the body starts going through some changes, all of which mean we can face physical changes such as reduced muscles strength, inflexibility, stiff joints, reduced bone density, and reduced balance. These consequence can increase our risk of falling, of illness, and of pain. Yet, whilst ageing is a natural process – one which is inevitable – the consequence of immobility are far from fate. Happily, for most of us, we gain wisdom and many other beneficial traits as we age. And so, we can understand that we can combat some of the negative side effects of ageing simply by remaining active and keeping on top of fitness. And besides, exercise can be fun!

According to the National Health Service guidelines (NHS), adults from 19 to 60 and beyond should complete moderate intensity, physical exercise for a least 150 minutes a week, or alternately, should complete 75 minutes of high intensity physical exercise. The activity should include cardiovascular exercises –"cardio" is heart and "vascular" means blood. This type of activity gently challenges your muscles and works the blood vessels so as to get fitter and stronger.

If you're reading this and thinking, wait a minute, Nash... I'm not a running, stop right there. It's not about running a marathon or completing in an Iron Man race! Cardiovascular exercises include brisk walking, swimming cycling, yoga/Pilates, dancing, and gardening. Unless you're competing in the Chelsea Flower Show, there really isn't any sort of time-based completion, here. You do what you can, for you, at your pace, in order to reap the benefits.

In addition to cardio, however, it is also important to include strength activities such as weight training, carrying heavy loads, and doing some heavy gardening that involves all major muscle groups such as legs, hips, back, core muscles, shoulders, and arms. Again, it's not about getting a six pack or looking like Barbie or Ken; it's about getting stronger, more able to stave of injury, and being more stable on your feet. Not to mention, of course, that these types of activities can be productive and fit easily into your day.

For women, in particular, strength training is very important; it encourages strong bone density throughout life. Interesting, hormonal changes in women mean that their bones and skeletons may become weak, s exercise such as this can, in fact, help with the regulation of hormones. Very often, the female skeleton endures strain as it is subject to changes in ligaments and bone strength which begin at puberty and continue throughout life – countering this change with strength training can make the world of difference. On top of this, carrying children and the eventual menopause are further catalysts for the potential deterioration of strength – so, strength training can only be a good thing, right?

Hormonal contraception is also a factor in the surging and falling hormones, which can eventually be detrimental to health. And let me take a second here to say that yes, it may sound like a minefield, but one sure way of winning against the tidal wave of change throughout life is to exercise – strength training and cardio are the best tools you have against some of the more negative effects of ageing.

And one more thing that I know is nice to hear is that exercise helps with weight control. Yes, a large part of weight loss is fought in the kitchen, but without muscle, weight loss cannot really be sustained. Muscles are powerhouses and need the energy from calories to function... the more muscles you have, the more calories you Burn!

And for women, in particular, it is important to know that fat contains estrogen, and, therefore, excess weight or poor management of weight can put women at risk of health complications – exercise will help stave this off. In later life, maintaining strength alongside weight management is vitally important. Estrogen drops post menopause, thus the chances of diseases like osteoporosis increase. As such, remaining strong is crucial.

Whilst weight control is a good thing, and strength is even better, there is an even more important reason as to why exercise should be a priority in your life. You see, as we age our propensity to succumb to diseases such as dementia, type 2 diabetes, depression, and heart disease increased. Exercise can, in fact, steer you away from these scenarios.

You might wonder exercise and disease can be linked, but it is proven that repetitive movement improves neuroplasticity (the ability of your brain to process changes etc.) and brain synapse reactions (messages in the brain), both of which are linked to alertness, functionality, and articulacy. I'm not saying that exercise is going to help you write the next great speech, but what I am saying is that it will give you more time to live the life you're meant to.

 The really heart-breaking thing about our society is that the above mentioned diseases are driven by an overarching focus on sedentary lifestyles. Older people are spending more time maintaining lifestyles filled with TV, sofas, and staring out of the window. They need to move. They need to walk, paint, pick flowers, and see their loved ones. The fact that activities for the retired population traditionally revolve around catching up with television or socialising in the pub should really be one of our nation's welfare priorities – this absolutely needs to change.

The reduced level of activity as seen in the older population may result in affected normal daily activities. Yes, that's right, it's not just about dementia or diabetes. Leisure activities will suffer, conversations with family members will be cut short, and mobility issues will result in the loss if independence. When this happen, most people start to shut down: they get stiff and then old, rather than old and then stiff. If you're heading down this path, the reality is that you might start getting aches and pains in your joints/muscles that you never experienced before; you'll soon have reduced exercise tolerance, reduced energy, and your balance will suffer therefore resulting in high risk of falling. You'll age before your time. You have to make the choice to change.

Phew – I think it's pretty clear that a life without exercise will soon result in no life at you're your best life is filled with movement, mobility, and exercise. I promise. Enough of the doom and gloom, though – let's get into the positive stuff. Why is exercise good, what can it do for you, right now, and why should you get those walking shoes laced up? Right after you read this book, of course....

Well, I constantly tell all my patients that an increase in exercise will:

1. Improve muscle strength/flexibility
2. Minimise muscle/joint pain
3. Manage blood sugars
4. Reduce body fat percentage
5. Improve mental wellbeing

Sounds pretty good, right? That's because it is! Nearly every single ailment can be better by incorporating exercise into your day: from high blood pressure, through to diabetes and back pain, exercise is a must. Exercise benefits the whole body, inside and out, and happily there are many more ways in which to exercise than you think!

## Improving muscles Strength/Flexibility

Our muscles are attached to bones/skeleton via tendons and ligaments; these ligaments attach bone to bone and allow us to move the body freely, all so that we can complete our tasks successfully and instinctually. Yet, what happens when this is no longer the case? What happens when we struggle to bend down to tie our shoelaces, or we find it difficult getting up out of bed?

Life becomes really difficult as flexibility and mobility decrease.

You see, flexibility allows the joints to move freely without restriction or pain through a wide range of motions. As we lose strength due to sedentary lifestyles, flexibility is affected and, in turn, increase the chances of injury, not to mention the fact that we lose out on many aspects of our otherwise active lives.

And so this fact, quite apart from anything else, is why we should be stretching daily and doing activities such as yoga, Thai-Chi, or Pilates. All of this can help us maintain the flexibility we need in order to complete day-to-day activities without pain. Flexibility also allows you to strengthen your muscles more readily – it's a mutually beneficial relationship. The great news is that some of our basic activities, like walking, going up and down stairs, shopping, and socialising with grandchildren can contribute to strength and flexibility, BUT, and this is a big but… you do need to put work in in order to maintain your ability to do those activities. The truth is, as we age the privilege of doing these activities without issues comes under attack. Remember, the body is designed to degenerate eventually; the day we're born we begin to die. Dark, but true! It happens slowly, but it happens none-the-less. How you tackle this problem, however, makes all the difference in the world.

Despite the doom and gloom of ageing, there is a lot to be incredibly thankful for. Some of our best years are lived after we hit 45 – with memories being made day in and day out. Nothing in life is a death-sentence; your attitude to changing circumstances, and your commitment to health, is what sets you apart from the rest.

You see, we can slow the ageing process down by maintaining an active lifestyle and eating a balanced diet. So, whilst you certainly will age, you definitely don't need to succumb to some of time's more negative side effects.

## Minimise Muscles/Joint Pain – Bespoke Exercise Plan

So, flexibility is key, but what about when it comes to muscles pain? Can exercise help then?

Well, from the day we are born our muscles, including the heart, begin to function constantly, without a break, until we die. That's incredible, isn't it? Do you know of anything else that can do that? Yet despite the incredible miracle of the body's function it, like many other well-oiled machines, run into one or two problems sometimes. It is inevitable to pick up injuries and stiffness at some point in the circle of life. General body aches such as lower back, knee, shoulder, neck, and foot ankle pain, to name but a few, are inevitable physical issues that we may encounter.

So, I believe the question is not really how to avoid them, but how to manage them. Medicated isn't the answer – that can be addictive and dangerous. There has to be another way… and indeed, there is! Exercise!

Now, the reasons behind injuries are endless, yet it seems to me that many management strategies tend to be generic. Why is that? You're an individual and thus your exercise routine should reflect that, right?
In short… one size does not fit all, and we all have different bodies, therefore we all should receive bespoke treatment.

Bespoke rehabilitation exercises, which are provided by a health professional, is one of the key treatments we can receive to restore health.

You might be thinking that this seems a bit of a stretch, especially considering I just told you there are inevitable bumps in the road, so how can these programs help, right? Well, let me explain; I'll use knee pain as an example. There are number of reasons why you might have knee pain, but for arguments sake let us say the knee pain is caused by muscle tightness and there is nothing sinister and no internal damage.

Now, without completing any exercises whatsoever, your knee is still vulnerable to re-injury if the muscles around the knee remain weak/stiff, even after hands-on treatment has taken care of the immediate pain. In other words, weakness of the knee muscles cannot protect the ligaments and internal structures in that state. Only bespoke exercise related to that particular problem can strengthen the correct muscles successfully – if this isn't done, injury is once again just around the corner.

And that is precisely the reason why physical therapy treatment should include bespoke exercises: it will strengthen muscles that otherwise could cause one to be prone to injury in the future. A bespoke exercise plan is truly non-negotiable, particularly when you're being treated for a wear-and-tear injury. Please remember this.

## Control Blood Sugars

Exercise and blood sugar... a match made in heaven! Most of us live such sedentary lifestyles that exercise is almost a misnomer. In our time, we see the number of adults over the age of 45 being diagnosed with type 2 diabetes souring, and sadly a lack of exercise is one of the biggest contributors of this.

You see, type 2 diabetes is when you have high level of glucose (sugar) in the blood, all of which is due to lack of insulin production in the body; sometimes the body also doesn't use the available insulin properly. In either case, blood sugar levels and insulin usage/production no longer interact normally. The long term effects of type 2 diabetes can be truly devastating. Problems with the eyes, kidneys, blood pressure, and heart are a few of the consequences. From limb loss through to nerve damage, type 2 diabetes is a killer.

Type 2 is not to be confused with type 1 diabetes, however. Type 1 diabetes occurs when your own body cannot produce adequate insulin to control blood glucose levels. This is not diet related, but rather it is an immune disorder. You see, insulin is like a buffer that helps the body break down sugar in the blood. Not enough of it and things can go from bad to worse quite rapidly. For this reason, type 1 diabetics remain on medication for their entire lives – this cannot change.

Type 2 diabetes, on the other hands, whilst is can be a lifelong condition, there is hope of alleviating its side effects. A holistic approach to treatment, including a change in diet, exercise, use of medication, and regular check-ups to monitor the sugar levels, can all make a difference.
The one I want to focus on, however, is... yes, you guessed it... exercise. How can exercise really help diabetics regulate their blood sugar levels?

Well, when we exercise we use the muscles in the body to burn off the sugar in the bloodstream. Did you know that? Exercise requires energy, all of which can be found in excess blood sugar levels if needed. Doing this means there is less of a need for insulin to breakdown the sugars on its own, thereby helping the body regulate the amount the sugar in the blood.

The flip side of the coin is a little darker, though. If we do not exercise, then inadequate insulin levels will result in an unsuccessful breakdown of sugars, thereby increasing the risk of heart disease, stroke, and weight gain. In addition, arteries will get blocked, thereby causing a whole other can of worms to be opened. You see, arteries are blood vessels that carry oxygen-rich blood at a very fast speed away from the body to the muscles. F blood sugar levels are high for prolonged periods of times, arteries get blocked, oxygen cannot travel to restricted areas, and nerve damage, gangrene, and amputation may follow. A scary thought!

Diabetes is the scourge of our modern society, and with obesity-related illness on the rise, high blood sugar levels may well cause the collapse of our healthcare system. Children as young as 4 years old are now victims of this disease... 4. Something has to be done.

Exercise is a great step in the right direction. When we exercise regularly, we naturally maintain healthy levels of blood sugars and reduce the risk of developing heart disease.

So, this should help explain why type 2 diabetes can be managed with exercise. Coupled with a nutritious diet, exercise can go a long way to regulating sugar level in your blood. It's just up to you to find something manageable, that is, some type of exercise that fits into your lifestyle and doesn't feel like a chore. They key is to fall in love with the activity you choose. The secret to regular exercise is trying out different things, even if they may be new to you. Remember, there will be time when the days we most need to move are the days when we least feel like it, and whilst rest and recovery is important, building up the habit of regular exercise is vital.

Many people make new friends and learn different skills through their pursuit of exercise, so it is additionally healthy for the body and soul. If you're put off by starting something new, just think about the fact that everyone has been there and that new experiences are fulfilling at any age! Also, you're doing it for all the right reasons: to prolong your life and maintain fitness. If you find something interesting, the time will pass quickly... and you may even find yourself doing more than the required level! Make the decision to choose life – don't let high blood sugar levels steal this gift you've been given.

## Reduce Body Fat Percentage

It's no secret that if, we exercise regularly and eat a balanced diet, we will drop pounds of fat. And, of course, this is one of the great benefits of exercising. Now, I'm going to be a little controversial, here... fat isn't all bad.

In fact, fat is actually very important to keep the body functioning well. Yes, fat isn't always a bad word, and it's important not to demonise foods due to their fat content. Remember, we all need a treat to keep us on track now and again!

That, however, doesn't mean we need to watch our weight – a healthy weight helps stave off disease and helps keep you out of injury's way. The key to a balanced diet is moderation, variety, and planning. Keeping track of what you eat allows you to identify problem areas or cut out mindless snacking, all so that you can eat in a way that fuels your body rather than hinders it.

We need to consume approximately 30-35% of predominantly unsaturated fat a day, making sure to keep the consumption of saturated fats – found in junk food such as chocolate, crisps and cakes – to a minimum. Good fats play an important role in the body, with one of their functions being the ability to provide energy for exercise. In the initial stages exercise, your body uses carbohydrates as the main source of energy. However, approximately 20-30 minutes into exercise the body begins to use its fat stores as energy. Hence, if you want to lose weight, then prolonged cardiovascular exercises – such as long-distance walking or cycling – is recommended.

Please also keep in mind that you cannot 'target' fat-loss. It is common for diet programs and gimmick supplements to claim that they 'target belly fat' etc., however, it really isn't as straight forward as that. Overall cardio vascular exercise helps to shift fat from all areas. If you're tempted to do sit ups for your middle, or undertake a particular glutes program, you will see some results there, but they might not be obvious.
If your intention is simply to raise your heart rate for a start, well, you can't go too far wrong. Anything else more specialised can come in time! More on this in a later chapter.

Unsaturated fats typically found in nuts and seeds also lower cholesterol levels and reduce risk the risk of developing heart disease. Think about avocados, olives, nuts, seeds, and fatty fish – how could you add them to your daily diet as snacks or healthy meals? The little changes may well make the biggest difference.

## Improve Mental Wellbeing

As I briefly mentioned in chapter 4, endorphins are natural hormones released in the body during activities such as exercise. Believe it or not, the chemical structure of endorphins is very similar to morphine! So rally, your body has the ability to produce its own morphine. Isn't that amazing? In-fact if you break down the word itself, the etymology points to the secretion of endorphins as a natural painkiller. "Endo", which means endogenous (having internal cause or origin), and "orphin", which relates to words like 'morphine' and describes opioid like effects, come together to give us endorphin.

Why mention all of this? Well, exercise should be one of the first natural interventions recommended to fight off anxiety and depression, even before pharmaceutical methods. I'm not saying it's a cure-all, and mental illness is very serious, but it is a good starting point.

From a more technical standpoint, the part of the brain called the pituitary gland can release natural pain killers through exercise, all of which, in turn, helps us to feel happy and create a natural high. This makes it easier to manage the symptoms and effects of anxiety and depression.

What about when it comes to ageing? As we age, our skin gets a little less elastic and we may not look quite as spritely as we did when we were 20, but for all the cosmetic imperfections, endorphins may actually have an answer! Whilst endorphins might not be as immediately effective as Botox when it comes to keeping you looking young, there is non-the-less evidence that shows endorphins can certainly help to keep us looking young and fresh. Why? New tissue is produced with regular exercise.

So, you look better... thus feel better, too! In general, exercise is great at helping you prepare for the effects of ageing and to encourage the body to keep on operating at its best! The heart muscles also benefit from endorphins, as the risk of heart attacks and other cardiovascular diseases is reduced. One can't help but feel good about that, right?

As I write this book, it is clear to me that the Covid-19 pandemic has severely affected the mental health of many individuals, particularly the elderly and vulnerable. The main contributing factor to this is, I believe, the fact that the gyms and health facilities have been closed. Additionally, we were only allowed one hour of outdoor exercise a day to get our endorphin boost. It very sad to see many people, including myself, feel stress, loneliness, and the fear of the unknown. This unique situation really created panic, and with routine and daily habits changing forever, many found it hard to stay on top of exercise. Many people were lead by their emotions.

That said, it was also a time for some to discover exercise, spending time at home, and finding out how the new routine was able to help them create new habits. Not knowing when things would resume back to normal, and with the large number of lives lost due to Covid-19, the collective concern and consciousness about health prompted many to make lifestyle changes a priority.

So, despite the unprecedented times we are currently living in, there is hope for us all in the shape of reverting to the natural pain killers released through endorphins – we can use endorphins to reduce stress, anxiety, and depression.

Still, it is important to be aware of the long Covid -19 infection symptoms, all of which might contribute to, or exacerbate, anxiety and depression. Some of these symptoms include shortness of breath, chest pains, extreme tiredness, difficulty to sleep, and joint pain. It is important to reach out to your doctor if your symptoms persist. Long standing health conditions like this can cause frustration and can severely affect mental wellbeing. Here are some physiotherapy self-management tips to manage anxiety/depression, some of which may or may not be caused by covid-19:

Exercise is on top of the list, as you may well imagine.

Another method to help ease and manage anxiety is to practice mindful breathing and meditative states. Focusing on breathing helps to ground the mind and puts us back in control of concentration if done correctly. It isn't always easy as all that, but clearing out the mind is essential to mental and physical recovery… if you can master it. In a quiet and safe place, close eyes and imagine yourself on a beach with soothing music in the background. Whilst in this state, practice taking deep breaths for 5-10 minutes.
You will find breathing control exercise is very useful to reduce stress and anxiety.

Mindfulness is another useful tool to use as you pay attention to your inner thoughts and feelings, all so that you can reduce the effects of stress and anxiety. Doing this will help you notice what is actually playing on your mind and will bring yourself back to the present. Relaxing in this way also aids sleep, which is a time during which the brain and body heal.

On that note, adequate sleep allows the body to rest physically and mentally. It is recommended that you have 6-9 hours of sleep for the body to fully recover. The amount of sleep needed varies from person to person, but without it the body will struggle to function, let alone tackle illness.

Avoid comfort eating or relying on alcohol. Don't smoke, drink too much caffeine, or eat many sugary snacks, as this can increase your stress and anxiety levels even though these types of stimulants may give you a temporary "high period". Quick fixes like this can be highly addictive and can supply a false state of happiness which becomes harder and harder to attain, leading us into a vicious cycle of bad habits which shortens our lives.

Last, but not least, watch funny programs or listen to jokes that actually make you laugh out loud! Laughter truly is medicinal and it actually helps the body release endorphins. In the words of Audrey Hepburn: "I honestly think it's the thing I like most in the world, to laugh. It cures a multitude of ills".

If you want to find more about a personalised video based exercise programme for you or a loved one – to improve general health and wellbeing – then feel to contact us to arrange a free 15-minute consultation with a health expert. You can find us at www.t4phyiso.co.uk or email info@t4physio.com.

I hope this chapter has enlightened as to some of the ways to add movement and healthy habits to your life. As an advocate for health, and as someone with an interest in feeling my best at all times, I can honestly recommend these steps personally. It isn't always easy to balance work, life, enjoyment, leisure, and to maintain fitness inspired pastimes, but if you can find the willpower then it will transform your life. Imagine yourself after the exercise, the rush of energy, the warmth in your cheeks, and the vibrancy in your step. Think of the restful sleep you will gain and the joys of fulfilling the healthy appetite you've worked up! It may be that you take small steps towards your goals, but every piece of movement is something, and each day will get easier and brighter. Let's lace those trainers up today!

As we move into the next chapter, let's keep in mind the benefits of exercise for our wellbeing and health. We look at diet next – so, go grab an apple from the fridge, fill up that water bottle, and let's get chatting!

# Chapter 7

# What is a Balanced Diet anyway?

As I mentioned in Chapter 6, exercising regularly is one of the most important things that you can do to keep healthy and minimise most diseases. However, this is only half of the battle. Why? Well, every good sidekick looks up to a superhero... in this case, exercise is only productive if it is in conjunction with a balanced diet. We truly are what we eat. It seems to me that many of us are not aware of the fact that the outward appearance of body is typically the result of what we put inside it, with a few exceptions of course. Yes, that's right, his six pack isn't the result of eating a pizza 5 nights a week, and her glutes aren't because she's a bit of a chocolate fan... it takes work, and it takes restraint. And you know what?

A balanced diet isn't just about weight, either. It's about health. In this chapter, then, we are going to review the truth about diet. In what follows, I aim to eradicate some of the myths and misinformation out there, all of which can cause a lot of havoc and confusion. I do hope that, by the end of this chapter, you will have clarity on what a balanced diet is and, in addition, that you will have a basic understanding of how food is fuel, and what a typical balanced diet really is. Ready? Let's get stuck in.

The first thing I want you to remember, particularly when it comes to gaining weight and diet, is that calories do matter. I don't want you to obsess over every calorie and lie awake at night because you had a bite of cheesecake.
I do, however, what you to be honest with yourself. We have to be truthful when it comes to 'tracking calories' and what our daily intake is, otherwise you've already lost the battle. If the input is higher than the output, and you don't exercise adequately, then you might find yourself carrying a few extra pounds around. If you're aiming to lose weight, then there is only one fact to remember: you must be in a calorie deficit.

If you're looking to maintain your weight, however, then moving regularly and moderating your diet is the key. Remember, your intake of food and attitude towards that food will rule your outer physique and inner health. Developing this attitude positively will help you build a successful relationship with what you put in your mouth. So, weight loss, weight management, health, and even weight gain all come back to your relationship with food as well as exercise – keep this in mind as we delve further into the world of nutrition.

So, let me start by defining what 'calories' are. What role do they play to keep the body functioning correctly? Well, calories are actually known as kilocalories. What this really means is that one calorie defines the amount of heat required to increase the temperature of one kilogram of water to one degree Celsius. Isn't that incredible? Think about it for a moment – the power of what you eat is so evident that, scientifically, the manipulation of the energy you consume could in actual fact heat water. This is just amazing.

If you didn't find that particularly exciting, that's the boring scientific bit out of the way. Coming back to calories, the average daily calorie consumption stands at 2000-2500, depending on gender, age, size and your normal daily activities. Now, this may seem like a large number, but don't be fooled. Calories slip away incredibly easily! Just ask your stomach at 1am when you're staring at the biscuits in the pantry!

The truth is, there are many different factors that affect how much energy intake one person needs, but despite this, those needs are usually met with fewer foods that you may think. People chronically underestimate the amount of calories in foods. And this misconception is all too often compounded by a sedentary lifestyle. Here's some food for thought... the above mentioned calorie guidelines were typically implemented based on the activity measured during the industrial revolution. Think about that for a moment: not only were those the days of manual/physical work, which in turn actually burned most of the calories found in the food of those days, but they didn't have the ultra-processed, fast food-type means and snacks we can now access by pressing a button on our phones. A shift in the type of job roles undertaken over the last 150 years, as well as an increase in the availability of junk food and convenience food during the post war generations, means that the diet to movement ratio has changed significantly.

Considering what we actually consume these days, it's simply not surprising that we're overdoing our calories. In fact, without trying awfully hard it's not difficult to exceed 4000 calories a day! Have you ever had a stuffed crust pizza? Well, I have a feeling you'll understand what I mean when I say it's easy to exceed calorie intake!

And here's the real bogie: in the 21st century a lot of sedentary jobs, ones which require long hours and which are mentally exhausting, induce a lack of exercise tolerance. Prolonged sitting in the office, driving, and TV at home, means that the overall measurable physical output is very low. How many of your neighbours are taking an hour long walk a day? How often are you?

As a result, then, our caloric intake far exceeds our ability to burn the energy off prior to it getting stores as fat. Consequently, obesity levels have skyrocketed, type 2 diabetes is torturing more and more individuals, and mental health problems are becoming increasingly prevalent. Something has got to give!

On a personal level, one of the best things you can do is adjust your calorie intake so as to either maintain your weight or to facilitate a gradual weight loss. I saw gradual because I mean gradual. Quick weight loss never, ever lasts – severe caloric restriction leads not to fat loss, but to muscle loss which, in turn, will inevitably cause you to gain more weight back as your energy burning powerhouses have been depleted. It's far better to restrict your calories consistently, over time, and in smaller amounts. Slow and steady wins the race!

Life is tough – the pressures place on us all to be the perfect mom, dad, husband, wife, employee, or friend can really take its toll. All too often we don't make the time to cook well, eat well, move, and get some real mental and physical exercise into our days. Mental exhaustion and burnout can make it hard to find the motivation to exercise and eat healthily, but I urge you to carve out some time and make yourself a priority. Do it for yourself, your family, and your loved ones – make that change.

If we think about the 21st century lifestyle, what stands out? Technology! We can now set an alarm for the coffee to make itself in the morning, we can use our phones to start the washing machine, and we can even buy machine that vacuum our homes and do the dishes. What, in fact, do we ever have to do physically? I find this to be a little terrifying if I'm honest. We're giving away our mobility and independence based on convenience. Please think carefully about this.

And yet, don't get me wrong, the development in technology is great – from medical advancements through to incredible advancements in transport and education, we're very blessed. And yet, how good is all this for our bodies? We now have ready-made meals we can freeze, vending machines we can access at the drop of a hat, packaged shopping subscriptions with decadent treats delivered to our door, and dare I say it, take our menus in the palm of our hands.

And whilst I love a good Indian take away as much as the next person, all this convenience seriously takes away our ability to monitor what we are eating, how many calories the food contains, and how it will affect our health. Gone are the days where we know what goes into the food, how to cook it, and how best to reap the amazing nutritious benefits of the ingredients. Most of us don't even know what to do with a butternut! What would our forebears say? We have to get back to a life where we know what our food is, where it's coming from, what is contains, and what the nutritional benefits of it are. Back to our roots, so to speak.

To add insult to injury, most people wake up in the morning and drive approximately 30 – 60 minutes to work. They then park right by the door to minimise walking.

When at work they use the lift/elevator and avoid the stairs like a plague, all so that they don't exert themselves. They sit for 8 hours a day and only stand up for 30 minutes at lunch, to visit the toilet, or to get a drink. Then they sit and stare at a screen while drinking calories in the form of hot beverages; they eat biscuits, chocolates, cakes, or other stodgy snacks for a quick energy kick. I'm not judging anyone – I understand that life is difficult and desk job is one of the more challenging things to navigate. I understand that saving energy is sorely needed when crunching numbers and concentrating for hours on end, but I promise you that if your food changes, your activity levels go up, and you look away from that screen a little more often.... Everything will seem better, easier, more vibrant, and happier.

This cycle of filling up on heavy foods which send our pleasure receptors into overload, and then spike our blood sugars, is a vicious circle which is hard to get out of! It really is – no one said endorphins generated by sugar aren't addictive! It takes commitment to step off of the hamster wheel. You really can do it though. And the first step? What you put in your mouth!

## What should be on your plate?

Now that we have defined calories and highlighted some unhealthy habits many people fall prey to, let us talk about what you should really aim to be putting on your plate in order to have a balanced diet. Before I go on further, let me stress that I am not a nutritionist/dietician, so I am NOT going to give you the best dietary plan or a meal plan.

I am, however, interested in your health and quality of life, and so my job is to highlight the basic foods and the general amount that we should be consuming in order to maintain a healthy lifestyle. See this as a guideline rather than a rule book – you are an individual and, as such, your food choices are your own. What I would encourage you to do, however, whatever those choices may be, is to do what is right for your body long-term. Make informed choices and be consistent in your decision to maintain a healthy lifestyle.

The major nutrients required for optimal body function include carbohydrates, protein and fats. The micronutrients required include minerals, vitamins and water. You didn't think I would let you get away with thinking water isn't essential, did you? Yes, put the Pepsi down! Lists over, let's jump straight in and dissect these individually. I will help you to understand each component in the hope that this information will give you a solid, informed foundation for making your own nutrient-driven food decisions.

## Carbohydrates

Let me start with the most maligned of all foods: the humble carbohydrate. Carbohydrates, or carbs, are frequently talked about with fair negative connotations in society, so much so that they've come a dirty word. This is nowhere more evident that amongst vast groups of dieters, particularly women, who proclaim the benefits of Keto diets and the Atkins diet. Certainly, the media simply doesn't help. From unattainable Photoshop'ed body-standards, through to most ridiculous cayenne pepper and maple syrup fads, the odds are really stacked against our friends the carbs.

Truth be told, it's hard to pinpoint where this started and why the unassuming carb gained a 'bad' reputation – for all we know, it all just happened on a regular Tuesday.

Yet despite the negative press, carbs are actually one of the most important nutrients out there. Not only do they facilitate the absorption of many vitamins and minerals, but they also make up the lion's share of our energy intake. Why? Well, as you should know by now, I love breaking down medical words in order to get a true understanding of them. So, to help us gain a better understanding, if we look at the first part of the work, 'Carbon', we can note that it is one of the big six elements that makes up the human body. This should already signal this nutrient's importance. The second part of the word is "hydrates", which is an amalgamation of hydrogen and oxygen molecules; again, the body requires both of these! Without turning this into a bio-chemistry lecture, I want you to understand the intricate importance of this nutrient. In short, the six major elements that make up approximately 99% of the human body are carbon, hydrogen, nitrogen, calcium and phosphorus, three of which make up a carb! Surely that's enough to convince you that it ought to stay in your diet?

All things being equal, we should think twice before we cut carbs from our diet, as the body actually requires them for optimal function. This is so true that, if we don't have enough carbs, we can actually get a bit snappy. Mostly this is because we're running on empty and fall prey to being 'hangry'.

Here's the thing, though, whilst I'm absolutely an advocate for keeping carbs in the diet, I'm also well aware of the need for moderation.

For those of us who enjoy a burger at lunch, a pizza for dinner, and a cheese 'toastie' before bed just for good measure... well, those carbs may be overdoing it a bit. There is always room for improvement and too much of a good thing is no longer quite as good.

If all of this has intrigues you, you might be thinking what actually happens to the carbs you eat? Good question. Let me use the humble Jacket potato as an example – our nations favourite tea-time meal, second only to fish and ships, can clearly illustrate the journey of the carb in the body. When carbs leave your mouth they goes into the stomach to be broken down into glucose – yup, the very same... sugar! This is ingenious as it enables carbs to travel in the blood and be used as energy instantly. Any excess glucose is then stored in the liver as glycogen for later use. Now, at this point carbs can, in some instances, turn a little ugly. This may in fact be the point at which they earned their bad reputation... but, give them a chance. These excess glycogen molecules are broken down by insulin and converted into fatty acids, or they are circulated to other parts of the body for storage as adipose tissue. Aha – I got your attention. Yes, it is stored as fat.

When that jacket potato is too big, or you're eating your third one on the trot, your body simply cannot handle the excess of carbs... and really, that's when you start developing excess fatty tissue... you know, that little tummy that's been bothering you. If you consume more than the recommended daily intake of approximately 150-250 grams of carbs a day over a period of time, then you will gain weight. If you're not moving to burn off of that excess energy then things will take a turn to the heavier side. So really, it's not the carb... it's how much of it you're eating.

In summary, the major function of carbs in the body is to provide energy, act as energy storage, and to promote digestive health. I would urge you to select wisely when it comes to the type of carbs you eat, too. Guess what? Not all carbs are the same – some are quick energy fixes whilst others take a bit longer to digest and make your body work just a little bit harder, thereby allowing you burn a bit more of that excess energy. So, depending on how active you are, you should choose different forms of carbohydrate for different days: the trick is variation. In general, though, you should eat more healthy carbs, known as whole carbs, as opposed to processed carbs. Whole carbs are found in foods such as brown rice, quinoa, vegetables, and whole grains. You should minimise refined carbs such as white bread, sugary drinks, sweets, crisps, etc. Remember, not all carbs are created equal just as not all carbs are bad.

## Protein

Moving on from carbs, what else should be on your plate? Yes, I know you were waiting for this one... protein. Protein, like carbs, is another macronutrient required by the body for optimum function. Again, like with carbs, there seems to be a bit of confusion and misleading information out there – what is protein, what does it do, how much do I need? So many questions, so little time! The most important thing to know? Unlike carbs, protein does not turn into fat if there is an excess of it. And it is this one simple fact that makes protein seem like a hero when compared to carbs.

The major role of protein in the body really revolved around repair and the rebuilding of tissue. Protein can also regulate metabolic rate/immune system, and it aids in the transportation of other nutrients like vitamins in/out of the blood. All good stuff, right?

Now for some chemistry: protein is made up of amino acids and it can be found throughout the body in muscles, hair, skin, and many other. Unlike carbs, our protein intake depends on body weight. The daily recommended intake of protein is a minimum of 0.8 grams of protein for every kilogram of body weight... per day. So, for example, if you weigh 100 kilograms, then the protein ration would be as follows: 100 x 0.8 = 80 grams of protein intake per day. However, if you exercise or workout on a daily basis, then you can easily double your protein intake to encourage the growth and repair of muscles. It takes a little math, but the result is worth it.

The good news about protein is that it is excreted from the body if there is an excess present in the digestive system. That's in direct contrast to carbs which are stored as fat. For this reason, many people jump into diets such as Atkins, Paleo, and Keto. Hold your horses, though – nothing is ever as black and white as all that. It is important to note that long term over consumption of protein can result in an increased risk of contracting coronary health disease, gout, or even high cholesterol, all of which can really detriment your quality of life.

Like most things in life, protein should consumed in moderation. If you already have a clean – unprocessed – protein rich diet, then protein shakes/bars may not be necessary.

It is important to understand that increased protein intake helps with tissue repair to aid recovery, thus increases muscle bulk in conjunction with exercise, but it is naïve to ignore other macronutrients in favour of this single one. The body functions as an interconnected, well-oiled machine – no one nutrient is an island.

Sources of protein include meat such as beef and chicken, but eggs, beans, pulses, and nuts/seeds are equally adequate sources, too. So, in summary, protein is important to include in your balanced diet, but remember that too much protein – or anything, for that much – is not good for you.

## Fats/Cholesterol

How incredibly dirty has the word 'fat' become? Not only do many people avoid fat like the plague, but people are often judged for eating full-fat foods! This is mind-boggling to me. Diet culture magazines aimed at the women's lifestyle market perpetuate a false, negative definition of fat. The truth is, fats are very important, believe it or not, and they should find a 30-35% space on your plate.

Yes, that's right. Let me tell you little secret: fat makes food taste good, and nature in her infinite wisdom knew this. We are instinctually attracted to fatty foods because they taste good, in the first instance, but more importantly, because they are vital to a healthy lifestyle. Nothing is done by accident in nature.

The key major role of fats include insulation, supporting cell growth, regulating cholesterol, and providing protection for our vital organs. Now, let me be clear about the fact that there are good fats and not so good fats. Not all fats are created equal.

Unsaturated fats are the good ones, and these are the fats we should aim to include more of in our diets. Unsaturated fats actually reduce the risk of developing heart disease and high cholesterol, and they consist of uncooked olive oil, avocadoes, fish oils, and soybeans.

On the other hand, however, we find saturated fats. These should be avoided or, at the very least, consumed in very minimal amounts. These include cheeses, chocolates, cakes, sweets, cream, biscuits, butter or ghee, palm oil, and crisps. Always read the label on your foods – always try to make the choice best suited to a healthy sustainable lifestyle.

## Cholesterol

So many people trip up here… cholesterol doesn't have to be confusing, though. I want to clarify, in simple terms, what cholesterol is and what the difference is between the different types. Alright, let's start with LDL, that is, low density lipoprotein. This is the bad cholesterol – the one you need to try and avoid and which can cause serious problems down the line. The other is HDL, that is, high-density lipoprotein (HDL). This is the good cholesterol and is, in fact, an LDL fighter.

You see, the liver produces cholesterol; it looks like a yellow, soft, flat substance. What is interesting about cholesterol is that in one form it is a recycled product in the form of bile. Bile is not secreted from the body.

Therefore, what this means is that your body does not secrete cholesterol, but rather recycles it for use again. As such, high cholesterol is best combatted by additional insoluble fiber intake. Why? Because fiber binds to cholesterol for excretion. This means your body is forced to draw cholesterol away from the arteries, etc. to produce more bile. And voila – cholesterol can be lowered.

As I mentioned above, LDL cholesterol found in foods such as butter, palm oil, etc. should be reduced; it can clog up the blood vessels, thus increasing the risk of heart disease. The HDL cholesterol found in foods such as oats, whole grains, liver, beans, okra, and vegetable oils actually transports the bad cholesterol to the liver to be flushed out of the body in order to minimise risk of developing health issues. So, get chomping on that fiber!

## Minerals/Vitamins

These are small, but very important, elements required by the body for optimal function. Firstly, let me mention the importance of each vitamin.

A

In medical terms, vitamin A is known as retinol. It is typically found in foods like salmon, yogurt, milk, and in vegetables such as spinach, carrots, and green vegetables. The main role of Vitamin A is to boost the immune system; it also enhances vision and promotes healthy skin.

B

When it comes to Vitamin B there are so many types that I will not go into detail. I will, however, cover the benefits and food sources. Vitamin B plays a major role in healthy brain function, muscle tone, digestion, and maintaining healthy cells. The main sources of Vitamin B include meat like chicken, shellfish, green vegetables, and eggs.

C

Good sources of vitamin C include potatoes, broccoli, and citrus fruits such as kiwi and oranges. An increased intake of vitamin C is good for wound healing, the maintenance of bones, as well as cartilage and cell protection.

D

Vitamin D plays an important role in maintaining healthy bones, teeth, and muscle strength. It is typically found in foods such as oily fish, red meat, and liver. And guess what? Sunshine is also the best source of Vitamin D – that's why it's often called the sunshine vitamin. So, it's best to get outside and take in some fresh air as often as possible.

E

Vitamin E is found in foods such as seeds and cereals containing wheat. It boosts the immune system and promotes the maintenance of healthy skin and eyes.

K

Vitamin K helps with wound healing and blood clotting. It is found in foods such as green cereals like wheat, vegetable oils, and green vegetables.

Minerals such as potassium, calcium, and iodine are required in small amounts, yet don't be fooled: they play an important role in nerve conduction activity and muscles/heartbeat regulations. You can typically find them in foods such as cheese, fish, and milk.

Approximately 70-80% of the body is made up of water, so alongside your nutrients, vitamins, and minerals, I urge you to think of water as another essential building block in a healthy lifestyle. It is very important to drink 2.5-3 litres of water daily. Water helps to keep the joints hydrated; it also improves brain function and promotes healthy cardiovascular function.

The thing is, sometimes it's less about knowing what to eat and more about how to make the most of the limited time you have and put together a balanced meal. This can be tough! Having a busy schedule can lead to bad habits and our health can deteriorate as life takes over. Planning is therefore key to a balanced diet. Everything in life is about moderation, and so it's not about cutting out or banning foods, but a lot more about understanding them.

It is sensible to portion out what you have on your plate so as to ensure that there are complimentary items in the forms of a mixture of vitamins, nutrients, fiber, and all of the things your body needs to function.

If you can visualise each plate or meal as a mixture between carbs, protein, healthy fat, and vitamins, then you're not far away! And what about snack? Well, why not add some carrot sticks and fruit to your day? Nuts, yoghurt, and oats also come in handy! The combinations are endless and the choice really is yours. Try to eat the colours of the rainbow and listen to your body!

Hopefully this chapter has helped give you a head start in constructing your meals and making small changes so that you can feel the benefit of a balanced diet. Eating well isn't actually that complicated, but the marketing of particular foods, and the changing narrative around what is 'good' or 'bad' can make for a confusing topic. Just like everything else, certain foods fall in and out of fashion. So do diet plans, for that matter. This part can be put down to celebrity culture and praise for particular body types or shapes – I find this fairly intolerable, as we are all different. We are ever changing and this type of messaging can be damaging.

The main thing to remember is that it's what you put inside your tummy that counts! Your heart and organs need all the help they can get in order to keep you ticking over. Proper treatment and care of them will surely make you glow on the outside, too! Becoming reliant on one food, or becoming too attached to one diet strategy is a doomed plan. Why? Well, firstly, you will get bored, and secondly, the temptation to binge eat will be overpowering! Furthermore, by favouring particular foods you will narrow your intake of important nutrients.

Stop this by structuring your meals and foods around moderation. This is always the best way to go. Listen to your body! If you're craving a particular thing, think about what it might be that your body is asking for. And always remember to drink some extra water before you reach for the fridge, or at any other time for that matter. Quite often your body may be asking for fluid, but you're mistaking that need for hunger. Yes, it's true.

Taking care of these basics will set you on the right path to a healthy diet and the changes will start to show in no time. Your bodily functions require a mixture of things to work as they should, and even if you have a fussy palette it's best to find ways to rotate what you eat. Please check the labels and ingredients of the things you are consuming. There can be some sneaky sugars hidden in so called 'diet' foods, and low fat doesn't always mean healthy. Natura, unprocessed foods should always be first choice. Be practical, choose all foods in moderation, and set out your treat days. Once you start, finding new recipes and learning about food will be exciting, not a chore.

As we move into the next chapter, we'll start to come to grips with what it means to age well. Ready? Let's get started.

# Chapter 8

## Ageing Well

As I draw nearer to the end of this book, this chapter comes from a very deep and personal place. It is inspired, just like many things I have undertaken in my life, by my 101 year old grandmother, Matilda. 101 years... that's a long time to be on this Earth – and thank God for that, because I've been blessed to have her in my life all this time. As the matriarch of my family, she has had a great influence on my life and achievements over the years, as she has done for the other members of my family, too. As you read through this chapter, you'll start to see why she inspired the title of this chapter: Ageing Gracefully.

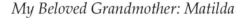

*My Beloved Grandmother: Matilda*

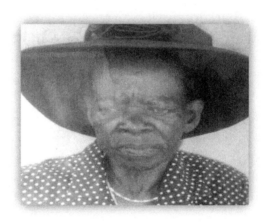

When you picture a woman over the age of 100, what do you see? In general, you might picture someone frail and wilting, right? It's not particularly often that you'd think of someone who maintains his/her faculties and lives a life full of enjoyment – and let's be honest, the sad thing is that there aren't very many of those types of people out there. Grandmother Matilda, however, seems to be the exception to the rule.

She is still very much alive and kicking and she maintains a very active, excellent quality of life. In fact, I'd venture so far as to say that her life is more active than most younger than her, let alone her age. She only uses a walking stick to stabilise herself or when she walks long distances, and, believe it or not, she has still not retired from working as a master farmer! How can it be? She seems to defy the laws of ageing in a way that many people are simply never able to do… does ageing gracefully, ageing well, perhaps speak of a deeper understanding of health and wellbeing? I think so, and I think my grandmother would agree.

Here's the thing: my grandmother is surrounded by her loving family and she only eats organic food, which all contributes to her longevity. Yet there is more to her extraordinary health than that: there seems to be a mixture of purpose and willpower working alongside the intake of healthy, natural food. You see, it's not just about the external influences… it's about a calm, peaceful, single-minded determinism to be both happy and healthy. That is the recipe for a prolonged and fulfilled life.

With our developed technology and advanced understanding of the human body increasing even as I write this, people are living longer and longer… and longer. Are people living healthier, fuller, happier lives, though?
You would think that quantity of life positively correlates with quality of life, but that is not always the case: even with all our advances, there is still a greater potential for people to develop chronic disease and mental health problems that reduce independence and abundant living in their later years. I think this is a very sad fact, and one which must be addressed.

A longer life doesn't just mean more time: presents new challenges to the physical and mental aspects of the individual, too. The mind and body can deteriorate in equal measure if the correct precautions aren't taken to mitigate the risks. Recognising that we need to take better care of our ageing bodies, and that we need to nourish them from the inside out, is a great way to tackle the effects of ageing.

This is something I want you to remember, as no amount of medication, Botox, or hyaluronic acid can ever substitute for a life healthfully lived. So no, we cannot prevent ageing, but we can definitely look at ways in which we can maintain independence and reduce the requirement for assistance, medical intervention, drugs, and chemicals. Happily, nature has the answer, and it's never too late to start making small changes which will help crank the cogs of our brains, joints, hearts, and more!

With all this in mind, I return to my grandmother: her life is indeed an inspiration, not only in light of her physical health and wellbeing, but also in terms of her mental alertness, capacity, and conviction. In my opinion, she has always been ahead of her time in her understanding of what looking after herself means.

Therefore, in so far as I'm able, I'd like this chapter to uncover some of the secrets she has shared with me over the years, all of which I hope will give you the tools and inspiration to really live an abundant healthy-rich lifestyle. So, listen up and pay attention to these healthy habits if you want to age well!

Let's get into some of the more nitty-gritty aspects of ageing so as to as truly understand what it means to mitigate the risks associated with them. We all know that we cannot be like 'Peter Pan' and remain young forever, but it sure is nice to be at least young and heart and pain free, right? You see, ageing is a gift if you choose to see it that way. Ageing brings wisdom and experience, as well as new challenges, and if we choose to accept these challenges positively, ageing can allow us to grow and live a fulfilled and content life. Our goals and priorities therefore need to adjust as we age. Rather than fight with the ageing process, we should learn to embrace and enjoy ageing well, as the inevitability of ageing is something we all have to deal with... it's how we meet the challenge of the years that makes the biggest difference. After all, life is precious and our main aim should be to enjoy every day we're blessed with!

So, let's begin thinking about the physiological changes we can experience as we as so that we can tackle them with the tools and knowledge needed to grow from them. The four major, inevitable, and most noticeable biological changes that occur with ageing are:

1.     Decline in aerobic capacity.
2.     Reduction in nerve activity.
3.     Reduced balance/co-ordination.
4.     Reduced strength and flexibility.


## Reduced Aerobic Capacity

'Aerobic capacity' is the ability of the heart to continually pump oxygen rich blood to all cells in the body, thereby helping us to stay active and alive. Essentially, heart health is indicated by how strongly it beats and, consequently, maintains healthy circulation. Unfortunately, due to the inevitability of the ageing process – which varies due to individual factors such as genetics – aerobic capacity declines by 10% every decade after we reach 50. Scary? Well, yes and no. You have the opportunity to meet this change positively and healthfully. Think of your heart as the 'bank' of your body, as it naturally slows the supply of 'money' distributed throughout your limbs and organs after the age of 50. The 'money' trickles through rather than rushing in! This means a reduction of 1% aerobic capacity each year, which can, if nothing is done, result in a reduction in quality of life and functional independence. If we want to get a little more technical, here, theVo2 Max capacity reduces. I'll explain what the Vo2 Max is below.

Vo2 Max, in simple terms, is the optimum ability for the heart, lungs, and muscles to work in unison and use the oxygen required to complete a physical activity or exercise. In this example, if the oxygen is the money, the Vo2 Max is how it is spent. From a sport science perspective, Vo2 Max is a simple tool used to measure and track one's fitness progress. It stands to reason, then, that if an individual maintains a sedentary lifestyle then aerobic capacity decreases accordingly, and the heart and lung muscles no longer function at the maximum rate. The more we are still, the more our functionality in this department reduces, the effects of which can be disastrous.

In short, if you are physically active in your childhood then you will be fitter in your teens, and if you active in your teens then you will be fitter in your 20's, and if you're active in you 20's then you will be fitter in your 30's… and so forth. If you are in your 50's 60's, and you want to be active and mobile in your 70's-80s, then it's never too late to start investing in your health right now.

You can begin reap the rewards of a functional, independent life at any time so as to reduce your chances of being unwell in your later years – being independent and mobile decreases your risks of becoming reliant on others. Your body should be respected and treated well: you reap what you sow, and what you put inside your body both via exercise and nutritious, will invariably translate into what is reflected on the outside. Remember, there is nothing more effective than a good diet and exercise – the negative effects associated with a lack of both of these can never be completely undone.

What you can do, however, is work to reduce the negative effects of past habits. I am no preacher of anything, but your body really is a temple and, as such, you should respect it and treat it well so that it can facilitate positive experiences and memories you will cherish. You truly deserve all of your golden years, because your health is quite honestly your wealth. Referring back to my grandmother for just a short moment, she has been able to welcome generations of grand-children and great grandchildren, and she's been able to share her life stories and advice with us all over the years: this is priceless and all thanks to her sensible eating and strong-minded attitude. In fact, her attitude to self-care, and the respect she has for her body, go hand in hand with her positive outlook; they both create the key to a long and happy life. As a takeaway thought, remember that, if you give up on life, it will give up on you.

# Losing your Balance?

At the age of approximately 45 and over, the nerve conduction system to decline. In simple terms, the body in covered in nerves controlled by brain and spinal cord, and unfortunately, as part of the ageing process, the speed of the signals passed on between nerves begins to deteriorate. This decline affects one's balance and coordination in turn which sometimes results in the increased risk of falls and accidents.

Located inside the head – in the inner ear – is the vestibular system. The vestibular system is a sensory system that gives the brain information about the movement of the head, general body motion, and spatial awareness. You can see how important this system is right off of the bat. In essence, the main function of the vestibular system is to help the body with balance and posture during movement. Can you see why I've mentioned it, now?

Despite the importance of the vestibular system, it is often neglected when it comes to maintaining a healthy lifestyle and ageing well. Certainly, as we age the vestibular process deteriorates and can affect normal movement and equilibrium. Does this mean it's an inevitable part of growing old? Do we have to be off balance and fall as we enter our later years? No, definitely not.

It is true, however, that we generally become less aware of our surrounding, and the ways in which we perceive our environments can be impaired as we age. Why? Well, the hairs in the inner ear start to fall out, thereby directly affecting our ability to gauge our surroundings accurately. It's odd to think of our balance are reliant on inner-ear hairs... but the truth is sometimes stranger than fiction.

We may see the truth of this strange fact when walking on an even surface… you might get a sense of the ground moving up and, as a consequence, leaving you disorientated and with an increased risk of falling due to poor co-ordination. This is because part of the system which signals depth and balance has started to wane. In the worst-case scenario, falls and accidents can lead to a fracture or head injury, thereby affecting quality of life and functional independence. This isn't something any of us want, and if you're reading this then I know you're willing to do what it takes to prevent such an outcome.

As I mentioned, despite the fact that the ageing process inevitably affects balance and orientation, the dramatic worst case scenarios do not have to be part-and-parcel of the journey.
The good news is that we can find and execute relevant activities and exercises to help practice balance and coordination.

As well as remaining at a healthy weight, we need to intently and purposefully strengthen our muscles. Doing so helps us steady our feet and will also facilitate a strong and healthy walking gait. All this takes practice, resilience, and commitment, but it's all worth it. Remember, a sensible way of living helps combat the risk of other conditions, too, thereby ensuring that you don't have ailments to contend with on top of a deteriorating sense of balance. Health is an interconnected web – one small improvement may exponentially affect your quality of life for the better.

## Importance of Strength and Flexibility

Between the ages of 30 and 80 we can lose between approximately 35-40% of our total muscle mass. Isn't that extraordinary? It is not unusual to start developing muscle fatigue more quickly from the age of 50 onwards, particularly when placed in comparison with your much younger 18 year-old self. You see, as we age the body becomes resistant to growth hormone signals, thereby resulting is muscle loss; this is worsened when an individual falls into a sedentary and inactive lifestyle. Resultantly, if left unchecked, this can result in a decreased quality of life and life expectancy. As such, I really want to place an emphasis on the importance of maintained strength and flexibility.

Stretching daily is recommended in order to maintain flexibility, that is, the range of movement for a given joint. For example, in order to bend the arm to eat, the elbow joint requires enough movement for the bending of the elbow to occur. As we age the joints start to become stiffer as joint fluid viscosity (fluidity) reduces and the cartilage – which prevents bone to bone friction – lessens in width. The ligaments that attach the bone to bone also start to become stiff, thereby reducing the range of motion available at the joint.

These changes will invariably have an impact on quality of life, and completing basic normal daily activities such as cooking, cleaning, and gardening may well become stressful, strained, and painful.

The type of movement we are capable of executing throughout middle age and our later years will change. Please know, though, that this is absolutely expected – it's normal to age. What isn't to be expected, however, it that we become entirely sedentary and dependent on others. It is vital to ensure movement is not altogether lost!

As I mentioned previously, the exercise and levels of activity you enjoy right now will go a long way towards the level of movement, functionality, and cardiovascular health you enjoy in your later years. The choices you make right now matter more than you're aware of.

## Why Retire from Work?

Let me start this paragraph by saying something slightly controversial... retirement can lead to an early grave. Why don't you take a moment to read that again? How can I possibly say that? Well, let me start with a caveat: there is a big different between your work and your job. I personally think I should not retire from my work, but from a job. You see, there is a difference between the two. A job is something that we do as an occupation, that is, in order to complete a given task in exchange for a fee.

Work, on the other hand, is physical or mental activity completed in order to accomplish or produce something for ourselves. So, there is a big difference, although work/job tend to be used interchangeably in many instances.

When we say 'work', what we actually mean is a little challenge, an output, or something creative that gives us an autonomy and purpose, a reason to be proud, a contribution, that is, something which you have to 'put your mind to'. Can a job do this? In short, work gives us purpose, as my grandmother constantly reminds me! And who am I to disregard her wise words?

So don't retire from your purpose, otherwise you might find it difficult to have a reason to age well. A lot of research shows that people who retire and don't continue at their job, yet neglect to carry out voluntary work or other activities are more likely to have a reduced quality of life and not live as long their counterparts, that is, those who are involved in teamwork and are invested in a cause of some kind.

From a physiotherapy perspective, then, 'work' is a form of exercise that ensures you continue to use your muscles to prevent decreased exercise tolerance and reduced health and fitness. This 'work' is also important for mental health and staying sharp and alert. Have you noticed that diseases such as dementia and Parkinson's are on the increase in our elderly population? Well, one of the major contributing factors for the development of diseases such as these is that people are living in isolation. This isolation, and the lack of mental and physical activities, leads to rapidly declining mental health and a much lower quality of life than I wish for you.

## Women's Health in Your 50s and Beyond

As well as general ageing, changes in women's health, as well as hormonal fluctuations, can add challenges to later life.
As such, the importance of remaining active when you're a woman is even more pressing when it comes to the impact physical changes have on the core muscles and pelvic floor. The decrease in certain hormones in females can make life more difficult for women, particularly those who have also been subject to childbirth.

It can seem daunting menopause really is – but, the main thing to remember is that your mental and physical peace is what's most important – changes do not have to be negative… you have the ability to embrace change so as to create a better quality of life in the long run. How? Well, activities such as yoga, Pilates, gentle step exercises, and even moderate weight training can help you prepare for old age whilst all the whole keeping the body and mind as intact as they should be. Growing older and experiencing distressing symptoms related to the menopause can cause upset and embarrassment, but if you can find the willpower to continue exercising, to eat well, and to maintain a positive mind-set, you will have the formula for an easier ride! For example, caffeinated substances should be treated with caution; there are natural alternatives and superfoods you can ingest instead.

Community is just as important and physical health. It is vital that you find similarly minded individuals who can support you whilst you go through these changes. It's generally easy to find like-minded people who run and attend exercise classes, all of which double up as social events to rejuvenate the body and mind.

And please remember to be kind to yourself during this difficult period. Your body is experiencing a huge surge and fall in hormones, and it's therefore natural to struggle and feel low. There is help available, and a healthy lifestyle plan, as well as assistance from your doctor, is a great defense.

I have treated and listened to many women going to hardships related to the menopause and I would like to tell you that, if you're a women reading this, then know that you're not alone.

As a married man I do think it's hard for women to feel 'seen'; many feel isolated and struggle to relate to others as they go through these changes. Having worked in the corporate world, I have noticed a lack of understanding amongst colleagues and it must be indescribably painful. I truly am sorry. Please remember, though, you're not alone. In the 21st Century there's a lot of new research out there related to workplaces helping women tackle the gap in women's healthcare; this research is addressing the negative perception of the 'menopausal woman' and I for one am proud to be part of this movement.

## Healthy Habits

As this chapter draws to a close, I would like to finish off by offering some healthy advice regarding physical habits to help you age well and stay active. Now, the word habit is usually associated with something negative, but habits can be very good things if the behaviours that are regularly repeated are actually good for you. One they're repeated regularly, habitually, they become part-and-parcel of your day and their benefits increase exponentially. So, here are my top 4 healthy habits… they can give you a kick start to a healthy and happy life as you age well.

1.    Avoid Eating Late at Night

It's no secret that our stomachs can be the ones in charge sometimes… especially at night and just before bedtime. In those hours the temptation to snack can grip us with a vengeance!

As hard as it may seem to do, it's important that you avoid succumbing to the temptation to eat during this time. Why? Well, eating late at night can cause weight gain and affect your digestive system. Those little chocolate biscuits come at a price. How can you change your habits, you ask? Well, allow 4-5 hours for the food you ate for dinner to digest; do this before you sleep, as this can not only enhance your quality of sleep, but your tummy is less likely to rumble as it digests the food – and for those light sleeper out there, this may tip the scale. Furthermore, brush your teeth a good few hours before going to bed – when you brush your teeth you signal to your body that it is done eating for the day… you may be far less likely to snack if you're all ready for bed.

2.      Minimise Alcohol

Alcohol is one of the most toxic drugs out there. No, no – I don't mean the odd glad of wine or your sneaky martini at the end of the week. When consumed in large amounts as opposed to moderation, alcohol can seriously harm the body… especially liver function. Whilst working as a healthcare assistant during my studies, I have personally witnessed people turn yellow because of alcohol abuse. Yes, that's right. Their skin and eyes turn yellow due to Jaundice caused by too much alcohol in the bloodstream. Needless to say, it was not a pretty sight.
It was humbling to see the damage alcohol can cause to the body and I truly don't want you to fall victim to its dangers. Therefore, stick to moderate drinking if you want to age well. Why not try non-alcoholic beer or spirits, or try some sparkling water and lemon next time you want to socialize.

3.      Minimise Caffeine

For many of you reading this, this is a difficult piece of advice to swallow. Sadly, caffeine is another chemical that should be consumed in moderation. As you may well know, it's found in the nation's favourite beverage, tea, as well as in coffee... the world-at-large's favourite beverage. Remember, caffeine is a stimulant drug that is commonly used by many people to improve concentration, focus, and to reduce fatigue. Now, there's nothing wrong with a little mental clarity, but the ongoing abuse of caffeine is a danger to the healthy ageing process. Moderate your caffeine intake by drinking more water, decaffeinated drinks, and by reducing your intake of soda. You'll sleep better, feel younger, and be naturally energised once you change this habit for the better.

4.    Cease Smoking

I am not writing this book to tell you to stop smoking. If you're a smoker, then I', sure that, by now, you know the obvious side effects of smoking such as heart and lung disease. You need only look at your package of cigarettes to remind you of the m. What I do want to do, however, is point out that smoking can prolong healing time if you do suffer an injury. Think about that for a moment. You'll be bedbound for longer, you won't be able to see friends, family, or loved ones outside of the home for longer, and you'll be dependent on others for longer.

Why? Smoking reduces the levels of oxygenated blood circulating in the body. This means that, if you have an injury that should typically take 3 months, it will take an extra 3-4 weeks to heal if you're a smoker. Needless to say, smoking certainly doesn't help us age well; in fact it might even trigger the early onset of the ageing process!

Now these are only my top 4 of the healthy habits… there are many other healthy habits that can help us age well – keep researching, keep being excited, and keep on striving to age well and live the best life possible.

If you or a loved one has any aches and pains, or you just want to take advantage of our free 15 mins health boost voucher, then contact us on www.t4physio.co.uk/contact or email info@t4physio.com.

This chapter was all about ageing well and gaining the knowledge and tools to give yourself a healthy jumpstart in the ageing process. As we move into the next chapter, we'll start looking at why physiotherapy may just be the trump card, and why focussing on the quality of your treatments can be the turning point in helping you stay independent and active. Ready? Let's get stuck in.

# Chapter 9

# Physiotherapy Treatment Explained

Throughout these pages I've tried to give you a run-down of some of the ways in which we can get injured, the areas most often prone to injury, how we can prevent these injuries, and how we can look at avoiding injury as we age. So now, as we are now coming towards the end of this book, I would like to chat to you about what happens if you have an injury – you've done your best and prevented injury for the most part, but pain seems to be creeping into your day-to-day... what then?

Well, the answer is simple: physiotherapy. If you don't know what that is or why it's important, fear not! In this chapter I am to give you a detailed explanation of the different types of physiotherapy treatments and why you can benefit enormously from them.

Physiotherapy is more than just a treatment after a rugby or football match; it's not solely for athletes or professional sports-people, nor is it only for the elderly or severely injured and suffering. The beauty of physiotherapy is that it is for everyone, no matter your age, gender, or profession; physiotherapy can improve your life in almost every aspect, and it can certainly reduce pain and treat the problem causing your discomforts in the first place!
You see, the main aim of physiotherapy treatments is to reduce tension, pain, and to improve flexibility, strength, posture, and exercise tolerance. Why? All so that you can increase your quality of life and so that you can do the things you love to do. Every single chapter in this book, every single tips and piece of advice, can be enhanced by the incorporation of physical therapy into your healthy lifestyle. Stay tuned for more information about this!

I would like to address a fairly popular question among my patients: what exactly is a physiotherapist and how does he/she differ from say a podiatrist, chiropractor, or osteopath? Great question. My answer is usually concise...

- Physiotherapists typically treat injuries or diseases using exercises, massage, electrotherapy and joint/spinal manipulations.

- Osteopath/Chiropractor tend to specialise in more invasive joint/spinal/cranial manipulations and organ treatments.

- Chiropodist/podiatrist tend to treat the feet, nails, bunions, and gait assessment/treatment.

Phew – many names for many things, but let's just focus on physical therapy, here. It is not unusual to one person to receive all the treatments above by all these different health professionals – remember, the care you receive needs to be judged by how. That having been said, though, there are a few things you do need to look out for when choosing a care professional: my advice would be to devise a proper set of questions and use your intuition to help you select the person who meets your needs most closely.

Qualifications are a foregone conclusion, but the relationship a professional forms with their clients, and his/her ability to understand the needs of individuals, is unique and very important. Know your needs and find a carer who is able to meet them in the ways you most require. When choosing a physiotherapist, for example, always consider how comfortable and centered he/she makes you feel. In my own practice I always aim to empower the patient, that is, to help them become an expert on their pain and problem in their own right. Not only does this making my job and their treatment easier in general, it also means that they will be able to maintain a pain-free lifestyle well beyond leaving the treatment room.

Before we get into some of the more detailed aspects of physiotherapy treatment itself is so unique and so effective. Where other treatments seek to eradicate the pain alone, physiotherapy really seeks to find the root cause of the problem so as to treat it effectively. This, in turn, ensures the pain dissipates and doesn't return. The magic of physiotherapy is that it aims to help the patient maintain a pain free, healthy, active life, rather than masking the issue and thereby facilitating its return further down the life. Painkillers, surgeries, injections… these are all pretenders. I love physiotherapy because of the very simple that fact it works… period.

Now, what do I mean by physical therapy in the first instance? Let's take a look at some of the more common practices used by myself and my colleagues to help our patients experiencing daily, debilitating pain.
What is Joint/Spine Cracking?
Some patients are not aware that physio's are trained to crack backs and joints in the body in order to reduce pain and symptoms. In general, these techniques are most commonly associated with chiropractor and osteopaths. And sure, it may sound scary, but trusting your physio to do these treatments means that you can set yourself on the road to maximum mobility and freedom of movement. And again, it is for this reason that it's best to select someone you feel totally comfortable with and to whom you can fully disclose your needs.

So, what are the benefits of having your joints cracked? Well, let me mention why your joints require cracking in the first place. It may sound strange, but it's actually a healthy part of looking after them. Due to many factors such as poor, static or dynamic posture, repeated tasks/movements, diseases, and injury, soft tissue such as ligaments, tendons, capsules, and muscles around the joints can get stiff and tight. As a result, pressure can build up around the capsules of the joints. When these joints and areas are manipulated, one may be able to hear a loud cracking noise: this is the sound you hear when there is a release of pressure and stiffness.

Just as your car requires a service to make sure all the bolts and machinery remains lubricated and squeak-free, so too does your body need some TLC sometimes. It isn't actually the mechanics of your body, that is, your bones and joints, which 'crack', therefore, rather it's the pressure and trapped air particles around them.

Let's use the spine as a good example of this. The joints of the spine are called vertebrae, in the length of which a very important nerve can be found.
This nerve, long and thin in nature, runs inside the length of the spine and is called the spinal cord. Due to poor posture, repeated movements, and general wear and tear, the ligaments, tendons, and muscles that support the spine can get stiff/tight. As such, they need to be gently moved – separately – to reduce tension. It is this "cracking" of the spine that helps to reduce swelling in the area e by encouraging blood circulation, the result of which is the breakup of any adhesions. Ultimately, the process reduces pain levels in the injured site. As a result, this leads to an extended range of motion and an improved quality of life.

## Gait Analysis

The word gait is thrown around a lot in the physiotherapy world, but what does it actually mean? And, why do you need to know? Well, both are in fact very important for a healthy, pain free life believe it or not. Gait is simply the natural walking pattern for an individual. So, knowing what this looks like can be helpful in treating and understanding the root cause of an injury, aches, and pains in the body. You may be thinking of a friend who carries themselves a particular way, or an acquaintance who has a particularly bouncy step. Essentially, this is their 'gait'.

If you revisit the ankle and foot chapter, you will recall that we reviewed in detail a normal walking pattern in order to minimise reduce the risk of injury. In truth, information gained from a gait analysis is crucial in the absence of an x-ray/MRI scan, as it can go a long way in helping to investigate the potential underlying root cause of an injury or to prevent that injury from occurring in the first place.

Furthermore, it can help the physiotherapist identify potential physical stressors on the body. Thanks to the development of technology, we now have specialised gait analysis machines and fancy force pads, all of which allow us to see how individuals distribute body weight during static and dynamic positions. The result? Better, targeted treatment. At T4 Physio we offer a detailed gait and posture analysis… to find out more, just visit https://t4physio.co.uk/physiotherapy-treatments/postural-gait-analysis/. Chapter 10 (the last chapter of the book) explores the importance of posture and gait so turn there to find out more.

## Benefits of Bespoke Orthotics

We produce in-house custom-made orthotics here at the T4 Physio clinic – as I mentioned earlier in the book –but, what are they and how do they actually work? Well, let me explain this by starting at the foot itself. Your feet are the foundation of the body and that means they are the connection between yourself and the ground you stand on, walk on, or run on. The play a crucial function in your overall health and wellbeing, and the stress placed on them throughout the day is considerable. It is not unusual, therefore, to traces aches and pains in the ankle, knee, hip, and lower back all the way back to the foot, particularly when we look at the foot as a whole, foot mechanics, and improper footwear. One of the ways to address foot issues is to utilise strong, engineered plastic, that is, orthotics, to go inside the shoe or trainer in order to give functional correction to your foot as you walk, stand, and run.

Think of it as a special mould to catch your foot, one which helps you avoid falling into unhealthy walking patterns which could ultimately lead to injury and pain.

The aim of the customised orthotics is to fit your arches perfectly. Why? Well, this helps control and maintain your alignment and foot-function. It also goes a long way to treating the muscle or joint imbalances in order to prevent injury and to give support where it's needed most: bones, joints, tendons, and ligaments.

In most cases, orthotics reduce over rolling of the foot, known as 'over-pronation', or they help reduce rolling out, which is known as 'over-supination'. They can also enhance performance in sports or activities such as standing, running, and walking by providing extra support to the arches of your feet – these supports act like spring-boards during activities. As your foot functions properly, the bespoke orthotic reinforces the correct position. The maintenance and eventual habitual adaptation of the correct position is best achieved alongside an individually tailored exercise programme created by your physiotherapist. As a result, the pressure on the muscles, ligaments, and tendons is reduced, and progression of the injury or deformities is often hampered significantly. In fact, in some cases you can stop the pain all together. Essentially, orthotics provide, a two pronged approach to treating pain long-term so as to fully improve your quality of movement.

If you require orthotics or accessories, or want to speak an experienced foot specialist to see if you need bespoke orthotics, please feel free to reach out to for a FREE guide. Alternately, you're welcome to book a free, non-committal, no obligation telephone consultation simply by visiting www.t4physio.co.uk/contact or email **info@t4physio.com**.

## Posture

Poor posture is actually one of the biggest contributing factors that cause muscle and skeleton aches and pains, particularly when it's not addressed properly. Why, though? And what come be done to achieve and maintain a good posture?

Well, I want to start tackling thee questions by defining first what posture is and thereafter defining the different types of posture typically present in individuals. So, what is posture? Essentially, it is the ability of the muscles and skeletal frame of the body to be in the correct alignment, all with minimal strain and whilst using the least amount of energy to sustain a particular position whether they be static or dynamic. Phew! It sounds a bit complicated, but it isn't really. The position mentioned here is typically known as the most comfortable position for the joint and muscles to be placed in in order to maintain a position or to move.

Now, you might be glad to know that there is no "perfect posture" we all sit awkwardly at times, and we all wake up with a stiff neck once or twice in a blue moon. In other words, if you maintain poor posture for a few seconds or minutes at a time, then it is less likely to be problematic in the mid-term. However, if you maintain that poor position for more than 15-20 minutes then it can become problematic, though seldom for extended periods of time. When we speak of poor posture, then, we primarily refer to the repeated, habitual incorrect posturing of the body, all of which can lead to injury and pain down the line.

Poor posture in sitting, standing, and moving increases the likelihood of developing aches and pains.
For example, if you're a "sloucher" when you sit down in a chair for more than 20 minutes, then this can cause strain across the lower back region. Consequently, if you continue doing this for months and years then you can actually develop chronic lower back pain. This is why maintaining good posture at all times is vitally important when it comes to minimising the risk of developing aches and pains later on down the line.

For instance, if your line of work is sedentary/desk based, or involves prolonged standing or heavy manual lifting, then it is crucial to keep an eye on your posture… otherwise you might develop some lower back symptoms a year or two later. And the frustrating this is you may not be able to pinpoint the cause – why is your back hurting, what did you do? Well, the answer is your posture – those repeated, habitual movement you made over the last couple of years have now taken their toll on your back. Now that I have explained what good posture is let me explain four types of postures that can be hereditary so that you can look out for them and correct them if needs be.

## Forward Head

Forward head posture is what I like to call the "pigeon" head position posture. In this posture, the head is positioned away from the midline of the body… a bit like when a pigeon walks on its legs and pokes the head out. This type of posture can increase tension at the back of the neck as the head is positioned away from the midline; the muscles in the back have to work extra hard to maintain that position. Forward Head posture is also known as the "text neck" posture, as most people nowadays are constantly looking downwards in order to operate their mobile phones – what this does is cause a prolonged forward head posture, thereby increasing tension in the neck and back. It is also not uncommon to observe the forward head posture in elderly individuals due to reduced muscle strength, flexibility, and increased fatigue.

## Kyphotic Posture

Kyphotic posture is also known as the 'hunch back' posture. In this position, the upper back – which is known the thoracic spine in medical terms – is exaggerated, therefore pushing thee shoulders and neck forward. This can be hereditary. In some cases, due to the ageing process and a lack of vitamin D, all of which can result in bone thinning around the shoulder and upper back, medical issues can ensue. A disease related to bone thinning in this area, in particular, is known as osteoporosis. In younger individuals, however, this posture can be caused by other diseases such as polio or by treatments such a chemotherapy.

## Swayback Posture

Swayback posture is an exaggeration of the inward curve of the back. It is medically known as 'lordotic' posture, whereby the hip and pelvis tilt forward and are positioned in the front of the body's midline. An easy way to check and see if you are lordotic is to stand against the wall and place your hands across your lower back to see if there is a big enough gap to fit your whole hand into.

If you are able to fit your hand in there then this can be an indication that you're likely to have a swayback back posture. If the swayback posture is not hereditary, however, then one of the contributing factors is prolonged sitting – doing so switches your core muscles off and tightens the muscles across your lower back. Other contributing factors include nerve conditions such as cerebral palsy.

## Flatback Posture

Last, but not least, is the flatback posture. Here, there is a lack of curvature in the lower spine, and this is typically hereditary. A typical presentation of a flatback is when the head is positioned forward, away from the midline, with the pelvis titled back, thereby resulting in muscles tightness and an imbalance around the hips. These muscle imbalance over time and can result in muscle fatigue and pain.

So, now that I have highlighted the different types of posture, what type of posture do you think you have? If you are have ongoing aches and pains then please bear in mind that it is important to consider where it's coming from. The source is usually the fact that you maintain certain poor-posture positions during your daily, normal activities. If you cannot figure out quite why you're in pain, how to correct your posture, or even where to start, please reach out to us. We want to help you address your longstanding postural issues, so feel free to reach out to one of our qualified, friendly physiotherapists here at *T4 Physio* for more information. Simply follow this link: www.t4physio.co.uk/contact or email info@t4physio.com.

## Electrotherapy (Ultrasound / Cryotherapy / Heat Therapy)

Electrotherapy can be used to reduce pain and encourage the natural healing processes via applying increased energy, that is, stimulating muscles by applying low intensity electrical current, light, sound, and temperature. However, the therapeutic effects of these modalities are short term. Despite this, however, they can be used in combination with other modalities for optimum benefits.

Therapeutic ultrasound and heat/cold therapy all come under the electrotherapy treatment umbrella, and they have the same outcome, that is, is to modulate the pain and reduce swelling around the injured site.

Cold, or cryotherapy, is typically used to reduce swelling as it causes the blood vessels to tighten, thus reducing the circulation of the blood. The cold sensation also temporarily reduces pain as it dampens down the nerve signals being sent to the brain. Essentially, this type of treatment therefore minimises pain in the short term.

Heat, on the other hand, works the opposite way: it promotes increased blood flow to the injured areas by allowing the blood vessels to widen. Heat also reduces muscles spasms.

With all of the treatments that are part-and-parcel of the physiotherapist's arsenal, how do you know which one to choose? Well, every time I get asked this question – which is often – I suggest that my patients use a combination of them to achieve optimal restorative effects.

You physiotherapist should always be able to offer different treatments in combination with one another so as to address a myriad of issues and to offer you the best chance of becoming pain free.

## Benefits of Acupuncture

The roots of acupuncture can be traced back to China; the fundamental principles behind this ancient therapy are based on a Chinese tradition which stipulates that energy flows freely through the body via channels. In line with this school of thought, acupuncture helps to restore the healthy flow of energy in the body and therefore to restore normal and balanced bodily function.

As a result, acupuncture – combined with physiotherapy – is now widely accepted, not just in China, but across the world. And although there are different methodologies in Eastern and Western acupuncture, the fundamental remain the same. I am only trained in the evidence based Western acupuncture, so I therefore cannot comment on the Eastern acupuncture. This latter practice is, however, considered more spiritual than the former.

At *T4* Physio, we use acupuncture as a complementary strategy, rather than an alternative therapy. In other words, it is used alongside other management strategies such as exercise and massage therapy. Acupuncture has been scientifically proven to be effective, but it does not work for everyone. As is true for much of everything in life, success can depend on a number of factors.

Of these, general health, the severity and duration of the condition, and how the condition has been managed in the past come to mind most readily. No two people are the same, and it is one of the strengths of acupuncture that we treat people individually so as to get better results. What do I mean by that? Well, acupuncture sees the person as a whole, not a statistic to be treated… and this in and of itself can sometimes make the biggest difference.

Acupuncture consists of the aseptic insertion of pre-sterilised single use fine needles into the skin and muscles. The needle insertion will feel like a mild pinprick and should only give temporary discomfort. Once the needles are in place you may feel a mild ache, numbness, warmth, or heavy sensation at and around the needle. This should not be unpleasant.

This is referred to as "De Qi" in traditional acupuncture and it is a sign that the body's inbuilt pain-relieving mechanisms are being stimulated. Minor side effects include some needle discomfort, drowsiness, and sleepiness following treatment. At times there may be bruising or very minor bleeding at the needle site and perhaps a temporary pain increase.

Dry needling is a technique whereby acupuncture needles are inserted into trigger points – tight sensitive areas in the muscles – in order to relieve pain and restore movement. Dry needling involves the same sterile techniques as used for acupuncture – the only difference is that the needles are focused around the tensioned area rather than placed where the pain has been deferred to.

## Massage Therapy

Whether you are injured, ill, stressed, or an athlete, there is scientific evidence suggesting that massage therapy is beneficial for all ages – for acute and/or chronic conditions alike. Some of the common conditions that are treated with massage therapy include headaches, chronic back pain, strains, fibromyalgia, whiplash, pregnancy, strains, and sprains. The therapeutic benefits of massage therapy include pain reduction, improved blood circulation/lymphatic drainage, reduce anxiety depression, reduced muscle tension, and enhanced joint mobility.

I think we have all, at some point, experienced how massage therapy can be beneficial, right? As such, it's worth considering this type of treatment as part of a regular self-care routine, that is, one that adds to your general health and wellbeing! It may seem indulgent, or a bit of a treat, but it can in fact help maintain a healthy lifestyle and promote better sleep, reduce blood pressure, and calm stress levels.

## Shockwave Treatment

Now, this might shock you! Please excuse the pun. In medical terms, shockwave therapy is known as extracorporeal shockwave therapy, and in simple terms it means pressurised air passed through the skin to the injured part of the body; this is done using a hand-held device that rather looks like a gun.

Less scary than a weapon, these shockwaves are not electrical but are simply pressurised air that can make a noise – they give off low energy sound waves in order to stimulate the healing process via increasing the blood flow to the injured area. Overall, this then speeds up the body's natural healing process without the need for medicines, injections, or surgery. In general, between three to six treatments are required, are to be performed at weekly intervals, and each treatment ought to last around 10 – 15 minutes; this is sufficient enough to reap the benefits.

The shockwaves are felt as pulses, and yes, this may be a little uncomfortable. Remember, however, that the treatment is delivered according to the patient response; if you are unable to tolerate the pain levels, the settings will be adjusted to reduce the discomfort.

You may experience some redness, bruising, swelling, and numbness to the area, though this should resolve within a week. This sort of treatment is usually ideal for treating shoulder, foot, and Achilles injuries.

## The Benefits of Physiotherapy Treatment

At T4 Physio clinics, physiotherapy is simplified into five clear objectives: promote independence/staying active, reduce the risk of surgery, provide 100% natural treatments, reduce chronic medication usage, and use lay terms to explain to the patient what is actually going on.

Staying active and independent is very important, as this allows us to do the normal daily activities of life such as gardening, DIY, shopping and socialising with our children/grandchildren.

Unfortunately, these mundane tasks can be threatened when we get an injury or if we have general aches and pains. The role of physio is not only to address the underlying problem by stopping the pain, but to also make sure you also improve function, flexibility, and exercise tolerance in order to exact the normal daily activities or whatever the health goal maybe.

Reducing the risk of surgery is a major goal for most people, as this comes with its own risk and in some cases. Surgery, whether big or small, has been known to correct one element and leave us with some discomfort/scars and potential risk of infection in another. Needless to say, going under the knife is not only a frightening experience for some people, but it also presents its own chances of things going wrong, as nothing is guaranteed in this life.

For example, as we age the odds of coming back around from a heavy dose of anesthetic drugs might be slim due to weary heart and lungs that have seen better days. However, this is not to say it doesn't have its place in medicine, because it does, and sometimes it is a requirement with benefits. At T4 Physio we just want to make sure that surgery is the last treatment option after conservative 100% treatment has failed.

So, what does 100% natural treatment mean anyway? Well, it means we want to provide treatments that promote and stimulate the body to use its own natural healing properties, such as endorphins stimulated by physical activity.
By the same token, natural treatments also give the opportunity for the patient to learn about their daily habits and take some, if not full responsibility, of the root cause of the problem, thereby minimising the culture of "the doctors will fix it for me". Another benefit of favouring natural treatment is that it reduces the side-effects and reduces cost, as some medical interventions like surgery and certain medicines can be very costly.

Being married to a pharmacist, I am constantly reminded that medication is necessary as part of pain management. However, what I do disagree with is chronic medication being used as the solution to the problem or to mask the pain without actually seeking or addressing the potentially underlying root cause. There are always a few exceptions where chronic medication usage is concerned, and this is largely due to complex medical diagnoses. It is sad to say that some people are always reaching for the cupboard for medication to reduce pain whenever it strikes and are reluctant to have physiotherapy (I hope you're not one of them.)

At T4 Physio clinics we take pride in creating patient experts, as we're truly persuaded that when we know better about what is actually wrong with us, then we are likely to do better to address it. I truly believe what we understand we stand under, and one of the ways to gain understanding is to create a learning environment.

I am definitely an advocate for exercises as I do my own exercises regularly, however I believe just handing out an exercise sheet without actually taking the time to explain the reasons and the benefits is not good enough.
That is why at T4 we take pride in promoting self-management advice and health tips to give you peace of mind and ensure the root cause of your problem is addressed.

To find out more about our service and how we can help, please feel free to reach us at www.t4physio.co.uk/contact or email us at info@t4physio.com.

So, there you have it: you should now have a basic understanding of the benefits of physiotherapy to help you manage your aches and pains 100 % naturally, without going under the knife, using chemicals, medication, or simply putting up with the pain.

We all deserve the opportunity to age gracefully and stay active, and there are ways to make the most of your life no matter what your age or the things life throws at you. As a physiotherapist, I set out to help people resolve pain and this grew into a passion.

That's why I opened my own practice and spread the knowledge and theory of physiotherapy outside of my workplace via what I do every day, and this very book is helping me do so now. Often, we don't realise what we have until we've lost it, and it's heart-breaking to witness patients who are suffering when all their pain can be avoided.

If they had been given the right advice and had been prescribed physiotherapy as part of their treatment, much of their discomfort would be a thing of the past. As I mentioned previously, my mission has always been to give my patients and clients full control of their health, to put them in the driving seat, and I want that for you too.

With all of the tips I've given you, and now that you know the invaluable benefits of physiotherapy, I hope you can me the decisions that count. We now move into the last chapter of this book and look at the feet. Why did I keep this for last? Well – you better keep reading to find out!

# Chapter 10

# From Head to Toe: How the body works together

I have saved the best chapter until last. That's right! This chapter is ultimately my favourite. Why? Because my favourite body part to treat is the foot, and this chapter is an expansion of Chapter 1 in this book.

Now, let me confess that feet have not always been my favourite body parts to treat; in fact, the neck was right up until 2017 when I was headed by BBC Strictly to give treatment to one of the dancing stars following a foot/ankle injury. I had to treat an ankle injury within two weeks of the show starting… I mean talk about pressure.

At least one of the perks, fortunately, was that I got the chance to attend one of the live shows and witness the magnificent energy and dancing moves that required the feet and the rest of the body to be function correctly. Needless to say, this was one of the most amazing moments of my life.

It was then my passion for, and fascination with, feet was birthed, and as a result I completed extensive training to learn more about feet in order to become a qualified and trained foot specialist.

A shocking discovery I found during my studies was that the entire body heavily depends on a solid foot/ankle in order for us to function correctly, whether we want to just walk the dog or get a personal-best in high jump. Take a ballet dancer or a boxer as a sporting example: they both rely on the feet to generate power and strength from the big toe in order to execute certain movements required in both sports. I am going to explore the benefits of having a solid foundation for the body, that is, having well-postured feet.

Our feet are precious and work hard for us, yet they can be neglected at times. Those high-heels and skater shoes may not be helping you in the long run. Neglecting our feet, and not taking care of them in the way we should, can lead to a multitude of problems in areas such as the ankle, knee, hip, or lower back. In this chapter, therefore, I am going to explain how some of the forces exerted on our feet can cause muscle imbalances further up the body.

I am also going to look at how the way we move can have a negative and a positive impact on form and posture. In the medical field this is known as the study of biomechanics, that is, a combination of the words "bio", the body, and "mechanics", movement of the body/joint.

The one thing we do as humans, a thing that makes us very much unique, is stand on two feet. Standing, walking, and running are all key factors in our daily lives. Mobility is crucial to our survival, happiness, and independence, and anything hindering our ability to be mobile needs to be treated quickly.

Our feet are the very grounding feature of the body – everything above them is affected by their performance and ability to bear weight. At first it may seem strange to link shoulder injuries, and even neck injuries, to the feet, but the reality is that pain is never as straight forward as one first thinks. It travels – and when I say travel… your foot may well be causing the discomfort in your neck. Think of your body as a complex structure, each part carefully balanced in relation to the next.

Individual walking styles are unique and can be influenced by many external factors depending on gender, occupation, general health (diabetes and other conditions), and weight and hobbies. Idiosyncrasies in the way we walk are natural, yet they commonly cause pain as life goes on. The good news? They are treatable for the most part! Enter biomechanics… an approached well respected as a result of its insight into holistic health.

Think of the frustration of an ongoing problem – one you expected to resolve a long time ago following physio, chiro/osteo sessions – yet you seem to keep having the same issue repeatedly. Pain turns into frustration, anger, and despair. And then? It all manifests in further pain! You might find yourself asking if it's your foot, hip, or shoulder… things can get confusing. Luckily, I'd like to make them a little clearer – let's break things down a bit.

## The Forces Affecting the Body

Biomechanics is a fancy word for how the body moves, as well as what the impact of forces on the joints and levers of the body is.

Now, then, I want to delve deeper and explain the impact of these forces and mechanisms of the body bring about movement. I promise, though, that I won't get too scientific.

The two major forces that act upon the body are internal and external. The internal forces include elements like muscle imbalances and skeletal stress on the bones, tendons, and ligaments. External forces, on the other hand, include gravity and ground force reactions. This means that the body doesn't function in isolation; rather, these two internal and external forces at constantly at play. In addition to these forces, we there are also other contributing factors such as lifestyle, job requirements, sport activities, and the environment we're in.

The body is constantly being placed under strain and tension in response to our forever changing environments. It doesn't take long for the body to intuitively respond. For example, the man-made concrete, fantastic as it is for us to drive our cars on, isn't ideal for us to be running long distances on. Doing so can have a hugely negative impact on the muscles, joints, and ligaments.

Now, I am NOT going into a physics lecture here, but you might be aware of Isaac Newton's third law of physics. It states that "for every action, there is an equal and opposite reaction". Let me put this into context. For arguments sake, if you weigh 100kg and you stand on a hard surface like concrete, then the group force reaction from the ground up the body is also 100kg. Alternately, if you stand on softer surfaces like sand or the beach, the ground force reaction decreases accordingly.

All of this means you will have less than 100 kg of weight going up the body, thereby causing less stress and strain on joints. In short, hard surfaces can start to affect the ground force reactions, thus increasing the risk of developing muscle and skeletal changes that can travel up from the feet all the way to the neck and shoulders.

Wow, I don't know if it fascinates you, but I am certainly fascinated. Another example of this chain reaction is if your ankles roll in and you have a low arches, it can potentially contribute to ankle, knee, hip/lower back, and shoulder discomfort/pain.

How does this occur? Well, let me explain: it is common for people to excessively roll in when walking; this is called overpronation. This motion is caused by different factors such as flat feet or low arches. Over time, the ligaments in the ankle become lax and therefore potentially lead to the shin bone moving slightly inwards. When this happens, it can cause pain in the inside of the knee. One of the bones attached to the knee is the thigh bone – called the femur – and that can also turn inwards slightly, thereby causing the pelvis to tilt forward in what is known as anterior pelvic tilt. Now, the pelvis is attached to the spine and, as it moves forwards, so too does the spine… and this is where mechanical hip/back pain can start. As a final kicker, attached to the upper spine are the shoulders – so, in turn, the shoulder alignment can be affected, thereby resulting in shoulder/neck pain. Bingo!

So, that's exactly why feet are the foundation of the body, and the impact from the ground can cause havoc up the body chain, often resulting in aches and pains.

Should you need a recap on the basics of the foot and a normal walking pattern, then feel free to re-visit the foot and ankle chapter. Here, however, I'd like to get into a bit more detail. The foot is formed by a complex set of muscle groups and bones, all of which work in a quasi-relay team in order to spread weight and take the load of the body.

Amazingly, the foot is intuitive: it will develop and mature so that your walking style, bones, and muscles respond accordingly over time. Sometimes, therefore, the 'wear' of everyday life can affect the very movement and function of the foot. As your feet mold to your habits, they can set off a chain of responses further up the body. Interrupting this process, therefore, coerces the biomechanical forces to shift.

Foot problems and ill-fitting shoes are common problems, both of which could be instigated by fashion or simple lack of awareness. It's hard to know what's good for our feet, and leading busy lives means we may just fall into the trap of picking up what looks and feels 'OK' rather than shopping around for what's truly best for our feet.

Poor footwear is one of the non-medical contributing factors that cause foot pain and bunion formation. In case you don't know what a bunion is, it is bony lump that forms on the side of the foot; it can be very painful as the big toes get pulled toward the smaller toes and forces the joint at the base of the big toe to be exposed to pressure from contact as we walk or run. If left untreated, wear-and-tear of the fat pad, ligaments, tendons, and muscles underneath the big toe can occur, thereby causing severe pain and sometimes limiting the ability to walk long distances.

This chapter is a continuation of Chapter 1 which covers the importance of footwear. As much as narrow shoes look slick and are trendy, they can actually squash your toes together and, if worn for long time, can contribute to bunion formation and other foot diseases. Another form of shoes that increase the pressure through your knees, hip, and lower back are... you guessed it... heels.

That's right. Can you imagine your feet having about ten times the normal pressure loaded onto them as you stand and walk all day in heels? Yikes. On the flipside, wearing well supported shoes will take the pressure off of the joints. And yet, if you're like me, I love wearing slippers, sliders, or sandals in the summer – they let your feet breathe and allow your ankle joint to move more freely.

The problem is, though, most of them do not always offer real support, especially in the instep or heel, all of which can weaken the ligaments around the foot/ankle and encourage the foot to roll inwards: this can potentially result in discomfort around the ankle, knee, and lower back. So, shoes matter when it comes to support.

These are just a few of the issues that can develop when we have footwear with inadequate support – foot disease and unwanted tension in the body are just the beginning. When some of the issues become chronic they can lead to early onset arthritis and severe joint pain. How can you change that, though? Well, the key is in looking after your feet. Let's see how:

## Custom Orthotics

One of the highly recommended treatment options includes custom made orthotics to support the feet by helping the arches, muscles, tendons and bones absorb the tension, and encourage a normal walking pattern.

Following the extensive studies and biomechanics courses I've completed, I have consistently been prescribing and recommending custom made medical orthotics to my clients. I've done this for a long time. Why? Well, this prescription has added huge value to my clients' personal quality of life and has increased exercise tolerance simply to complete normal daily activities such as gardening and walking the dog, exponentially.

And this is especially with regard to my 50 year and older clients, that is, those who are serious about protecting their health. Many of them have written fabulous reviews about how their orthotics aid comfort while protecting their joints, all without compromising on their favourite footwear! And the best part? They've remained active! Why not read some of their reviews here: https://t4physio.co.uk/client-journeys.

Before I delve deeper into how custom orthotics work, let me start by telling you some of the reasons why they might NOT have worked if you have previously tried them. If you think they're a just a pointless piece of plastic that goes inside the shoe/trainer, well, then you've probably had a bad experience and need help understanding why that simply isn't true!

Most people just buy orthotic insoles online and hope that, by simply wearing them, their foot pain, Plantar Fasciitis, or foot/leg pain will automatically vanish. It's not as simple as this, I'm afraid, which is why you need to be empowered with information before you make a decision.

You see, before you start using or prescribing orthotic insoles, you need to consider whether there is any leg length discrepancy. This simply means that you need to check if you have one leg slightly shorter than the other.

Why? Well, knowing this vital information will allow for the correct adjustments of the insoles to be mad. A trained health professional will accurately measure the actual difference and prescribe the custom insoles accordingly. When the custom orthotics are prescribed correctly, and when used alongside a bespoke exercise rehabilitation program, appropriate footwear advice, and walking pattern education, the orthotics WORK BRILLIANTLY. Please be aware that the medical custom-made orthotic will NOT work on its own – you really do need a specific rehabilitation program to adhere to alongside it.

Now that I have highlighted why custom made orthotics might not work, I would like to chat to you about what they actually are and how they really can work. Custom-made orthotics are designed to control alignment and the function of your foot, all in order to treat or prevent injury-causing force on bones, joints, tendons, and ligaments. Often, they are used to limit motions such as excessive pronation (rolling-in) and excessive supination (rolling-out). They also make activities such as running, walking – even standing – more efficient. What's more, they can act in way that redistributes pressure on the bottom of the foot so as to relieve pain from excessive pressure or calluses.

A true custom made orthotic should fit like a glove. That means, all of the inside, outside, and middle arches along with the heel should be supported. Remember, this is only possible when a laboratory receives an impression of your foot. Ideally, this would be created by using a 3D laser scanner for more accuracy. Please note that the knowledge and training of the health professional taking the scan is what determines the quality fitting of the orthotic. This is very important. Why? Well, the health professional will be able to share with the lab other vital information regarding the foot, particularly the information that wasn't picked up by the scan. Each foot is unique!

Avoid orthotics that are heat activated or are glued on, as they tend not to be durable. Furthermore, they may not fit perfectly and might flatten out after 2-3 months. It is important to ensure that the orthotic has enough rigidity to actually give the support required, yet they also need to be soft enough to give comfort.

It is common to have discomfort for 6-8 weeks after wearing custom orthotics for the first time. This happens your foot will be forced into a more natural or neutral position. After years of morphing into its own shape, the straightening-out process can cause some moderate pain.

Don't worry, though! In most cases, the reason for orthotics tends to be arch-related or to do with bunion formation, both of which result in an increased ground force reaction that can cause strain and affect the foot mechanics in the first place. The temporary discomfort of the orthotics is much more preferable to the long-term effects of this type of stress.

And remember, eventually your feet adapt to change, thereby resulting in much-improved symptoms and increased function. Now, one of the typical questions I get asked in the clinic is: "How long do I need to wear the orthotics?" Well, my answer is usually: "it depends on each individual". Some people will need them for life, especially if they have a nerve condition or inherited certain foot types/poor foot mechanics, and others might only need them for 6-12 months in order to restore normal foot function.

So, in summary, an orthotic is a corrective device that can be medically prescribed to help the muscles, tendons, and bones of your feet and lower body function without suffering from aches and pains.

When prescribed by a specialist to treat a medical condition custom orthotics not only decrease pain in your feet, but also address the underlying issues that could be causing knee, hip, lower back, and even shoulder and neck pain.

It is important to know that, when it comes to most things in life – whether it's buying a piece of garment or buying a house – one size does not fit all. It is insanity to think that someone can create a custom made orthotic to fit your perfect arch without analysing your feet first in order to identify your unique arches.

True custom orthotics are made only when a trained foot specialist assesses your feet and arches, and then takes images or an impression of your foot (we use our latest 3-D laser scanner at *T4 Physio*) to create a perfect fit.

This makes custom prescription foot orthotics the most functional footwear when it comes to controlling the alignment and function of your foot, all to either give general support for comfort, or treat or prevent injury by reducing ground force reactions to the bones, joints, tendons, and ligaments. In general, most people, when they stand, walk or run, tend to roll excessively toward the instep (inside arch), thereby causing various injuries such as shin splints, bunions, heel pain, plantar fasciitis, knee, hip and lower back injuries too.

Let me explain without getting too medical. The foot/ankle bones are closely linked together to form a natural unique arch that can be flat, low, or high. The form is typically inherited or, in some cases, is as a result of poor footwear and the environment the foot is exposed to. If you recall in chapter 1, I talk about the natural, normal walking gait pattern and the important function and anatomy of the foot.

Now, let me explain using excessive rolling in of the foot as an example of how this can impact the joint within and above the foot and ankle, as this is common in most people and it can cause havoc on the rest of the body if left untreated for a prolonged period. Now, please pay attention, as what I am about to say is very important and it might just be the underlying root cause of your aches and pains… and your treating therapist might not be aware of it either.

So, in general people are born with either a low arch, high arch, or normal arch, and in some cases the arch type may alter due to factors such as footwear, environment, and medical conditions.

Your foot arch is classified as normal when the arch is neither high nor low, but has a noticeable curve. It doesn't necessarily mean you're going run fast like Usain Bolt, but it does mean you're likely to have decent shock absorbing feet and you're less likely to develop foot/ankle problems.

If you're flat footed, you're very likely to have a flat arch as this means most of the foot (particularly the inside of the foot) might be kissing the ground every time you stand or walk. This means the inside of the foot gets closer to the ground, thereby reducing the shock absorbing ability and medial arch support (inside arch of the foot). As a result, you're likely to have increased ground force reaction going through the base of the feet, all of which can negatively impact not only the foot/ankle joint and muscles, but also the joints and muscles above.

High arch individuals typically see the footprint in the heel/ball of your foot and the toes. Inevitably, your feet can have an extra hard time absorbing the impact resulting in an increased ground force reaction going through the feet.
What foot type do you have? Have a look at your print next time you're walking on a sandy beach!

Your foot and ankle joint is joined together with the shin bones (tibia and fibula) to form the ankle joint at the bottom and the knee joint at top. Keynote here: your calf muscle (its the muscle behind the lower leg) starts from the bottom of your thigh bone, which means it crosses over the knee joint to insert into the back of the heel of the foot. This means the calf is a shared muscle and any alteration at the foot/ankle or knee when we stand, walk, or run will impact both joints and muscles.

For instance, if an individual with overpronating feet – rolling inwards excessively – doesn't get treatment, then this can potentially start to cause pain underneath the foot, thereby resulting injuries such as bunion and plantar fasciitis (heel or forefoot pain underneath the foot).   One of the major contributing factors to such injuries is increased ground force reactions that may result in unwanted joints, ligaments, tendons, and muscle pain. Wait! If the pain only stops at the foot/ankle joint, then you're actually one of the lucky ones because, if left untreated, the impact will start making unplanned travel up to the body. That's right – the knee is the next pit stop.

Think of the body as a long chain closely linked by the joints which allow the body to move as a whole. This is great. On the flip side, it's not so great if things are not working correctly for one reason or another. If the foot is rolling in excessively, then it might impact the knee by placing excessive stress on the inside of the knee.

I dare you to try this now. In a sitting position, place your left hand underneath your left foot and your right hand inside your left knee. Now, gently roll your foot in and out to squeeze your left hand while feeling the tension alter at the knee with left hand. You should feel minor alteration to indicate the link between the knee and foot. In short if you experience knee pain then do check out the feet to see what they're up to... the body never works in isolation; it works as a happy family. The unplanned journey may continue working its way the body, causing havoc as the compensation heads for the next pit stop... the hip.

Unlike the foot and ankle, the knee and hip joints have a lot in common when it comes to sharing muscles; this only means more things are likely to go wrong and, in this case, thanks to the excessively rolling in foot, the hip pain/injury maybe augmented too. Let me explain how this might be.

The hip joint is so strong that if you're a woman then you may have the potential to get pregnant and carry another human being inside you thanks to the solid hip joint. It is made up of the thigh bone, known as the femur and the pelvis. As a result, the hip joint requires back-up from the surrounding muscles, and the knee happens to be the happy neighbour offering the support. Without causing confusion by going into too much science, the thigh bone can start to compensate by turning inward towards the midline of the body due to the pressure placed inside the knee.

That's right. It possible to have knock knees, known as valgus knees, whereby the knee turn inwards which, in turn, causes the thigh bone to do the same causing pain/injury to the hip if ignored for prolonged periods. With all these changes happening at the hip, it is not uncommon to start experiencing shortening and tightening of the knee and hip muscles: this can impact our normal walking pattern and, unsurprisingly, back pain might start. Oh yes, I know… who would've thought the prime suspect for an achy back will be the rolling in the foot, right!? Let's continue, as the unplanned journey continues to work its way up the body; the next pit stop is the lower back.

The medical term for the lower back joint is the sacroiliac joint (SIJ) which sits between the sitting bone known as the sacrum, and the iliac bone which makes up the pelvis. Where the two bones meet at the back it forms a small triangle shape bone known as the tailbone. Now, just as a side note, it is important to point out that it is common for pregnancy related hormones to cause SIJ joint pain. The thigh bone inserts into the side of the SIJ joint to form the legs and the hip joint. If the inward turning of the thigh bone remains unresolved then gradually this may result in forward leaning of the pelvis known as anterior pelvic tilt, thereby resulting in tightness of the hip flexors muscle group.

At this point, the unplanned journey up the body continues: the compensation from the front of the body can potentially move to the back due to the forward tilting of the pelvis, thus potentially leading to lower back pain, SIJ joint pain, and piriformis syndrome (pain deep inside the buttocks). It is not unusual for further compensation to cause aches and pains in the upper back.

Wow! Amazing. At least you're now aware of how the body is linked head to toe, and when treating injuries a holistic approach is necessary in order to spot any potential imbalances and misalignment. Remember, foot/ankle injuries can travel up the body and can potentially cause unwanted tension to the rest of the above joints, muscles, ligaments, and tendons in the body.

If you would like to arrange a free 15 minutes with a foot specialist at T4 Physio to sort any unwanted tension and prevent wear-and-tear (potentially arthritis), then visit our website www.t4physio.co.uk/contact or email info@t4physio.com.

At my Manchester clinics, *T4 Physio*, we prescribe 3D custom made orthotics that come with a 10-15 year guarantee/warranty. We also have the latest 3D Orthotic Printer that prints them within a matter of 2-3 hours – that means you can walk away with them the same day! To get a FREE 15 minute consultation without foot specialist, simply visit our website: www.t4physio.co.uk/contact or email info@t4physio.com.

Now that we have come to the end of this book, I hope you have been encouraged to stay active and maintain a healthy lifestyle. I would like to leave you with a Bible quote that reads as follows:

Dear friend, I hope all is well with you and that you are as healthy in body as you are strong in spirit.

*3 John 1v2*

Thank you for reading, and I hope you are inspired to use some of the advice contained within these pages to make changes that will benefit your life and ultimately bring you happiness. One of the reasons I embarked on a career in healthcare is because I have had my own journey with pain and injury.

This journey has created a passion in me to ensure others do not have to suffer. My philosophy in life, and in work, is heavily focused on teamwork – what are we but one huge team? We are a community, a city, a country, a world.
If we can help each other with healthy advice then everyone becomes stronger, and the benefits of healthy habits have the opportunity to run deep. I want to reach as many patients as possible, and I can only fit so many into my day!

So, I decided to share my wisdom in the hope of reaching many others and their families as they grow older and look to enjoy life every day, whether working, studying, or retiring. I hope you've enjoyed reading this book and that its pages will be well thumbed and referenced by you! Pass it on to a friend!

Our clinics in the north of Manchester are community hubs; we have so many loyal clients who help to fill my life with joy, too. Health and happiness really go hand in hand and this is my contribution to that. Many of our physical ailments can cause poor mental health, and the reverse is also true! That's why it's important to listen to your body and put yourself first! Remember, self-care is not selfish.

Stay blessed and look out for my next book about discovering the secrets of avoiding 10 deadly common lower leg injuries.

Printed in Great Britain
by Amazon